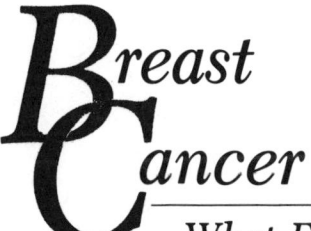

Breast Cancer
What Every Woman Should Know

Second Edition

Paul Rodriguez, M.D.

Aurora Publishing Company
Garden City, Kansas

© Copyright 1988 by Paul Rodriguez, M.D.

(All Rights Reserved)

Published by Aurora Publishing Company
P.O. Box 2537, Garden City, Kansas 67846

Telephone: 1-800-535-5111

Printed in the U.S.A.

ISBN 0-9622118-0-X

To my best friend, lover and wife—
My Delightful Nancy

About the Author

Paul Rodriguez, M.D., is a native of Arizona. Following his graduation from Arizona State University, with a B.A. in Science, he attended the University of Tennessee College of Medicine. Dr. Rodriguez completed his residency in Radiation Therapy and Diagnostic Radiotherapy at Los Angeles County Hospital and St. Joseph's Hospital in Phoenix.

Since 1971, Dr. Rodriguez has practiced Radiation Oncology and Diagnostic Radiology at St. Catherine's Hospital in Garden City, Kansas. During his treatment of thousands of cancer patients he has continually witnessed a lack of communication between physician and patient, particularly in the area of breast cancer. With this in mind, he felt that a book was warranted which organized the basic information and also provided an overview of the entire field of cancer treatment. The result was *BREAST CANCER (What Every Woman Should Know)*.

Dr. Rodriguez lives in Garden City, Kansas, with his wife, Nancy and children, Angie, Paul, Jr., Tina, Eric, and Roman.

Foreword

One day in April of 1989, a close friend, Judy Allan, who is a book designer, received the manuscript for *BREAST CANCER (What Every Woman Should Know)* from Dr. Rodriguez. That same day, she had a call from me. I had just learned that I had cancer in both breasts.

Like everyone else who hears this devastating news, I was in shock, terribly frightened, and very much confused as to what had happened to me. I couldn't remember exactly what the doctor had said, I didn't know the questions to ask, and worst of all, I had to wait. I had to wait for the tests to be reviewed, I had to wait for other opinions, I had to wait to learn the treatment options.

Sensing that Dr. Rodriguez would not mind, Judy immediately got a copy of the manuscript to me. It was the greatest favor she could have performed. Perhaps like you, I knew nothing more about medicine than how to get rid of a headache and until then, cancer had been the last thing on my mind. As I read *BREAST CANCER*, I began to comprehend what had befallen me, and what I could expect in the future. The book was written in terms I could understand and provided a 100% overview. I learned that although my family has no history of the disease, I had indeed been somewhat at risk. I am 42, have never had children, I smoked, and as a New Yorker, I live in probably one of the most stressful environments in the world. Although I am slender and an exercise fanatic, I would rather grab a cheese danish than an apple in the morning.

Since you're reading this book, I would assume that either you have breast cancer or someone close to you does. You are about to learn everything that you need to know about our disease and I guarantee that when you finish it, you'll not only be a mini-authority, you will have a much higher level of comfort as you enter the various stages of your treatment.

Next week, I will have a bilateral (double) mastectomy. After that, I'm looking forward to a long and healthy life because I was one of the lucky ones. My cancer was caught even before tumors had formed and thus, my prognosis is excellent. Therefore, I want to get the jump on Dr. Rodriguez and introduce you to a phrase that you'll read over and over throughout this book: **Early Diagnosis Is The Key To Recovery.** Dr. Rodriguez cites the fact that 90% of all breast cancers could be cured by early discovery so get your friends, your sisters, your mothers, your daughters, your aunts, your nieces and your grandmothers in for a mammogram. If they can't afford it, their local chapter of the American Cancer Society will advise them as to where they can receive an x-ray for free or at a sliding rate. And don't let them put it off out of fear of receiving bad news. After all, if a malignancy is indeed present, wouldn't they rather know now then hear the diagnosis after having postponed the appointment for too long?

Good luck and may you or yours be blessed with a full and permanent recovery.

Susie Kasper
New York City
May, 1989

Contents

1.	General Considerations	1
2.	Treatment Team	5
3.	Diagnosis of Cancer of the Breast	15
4.	Treatment of "Early" Breast Cancer	25
5.	Treatment of Advanced Breast Cancer	39
6.	Recurrent Cancer of the Breast	45
7.	Breast Reconstruction	49
8.	Anatomy	53
9.	Breast Self-Examination (BSE)	55
10.	Sex and Breast Cancer	61
11.	Risk Factors	65
12.	Cancer Prevention	69
13.	Chemotherapeutic Agents	77
	Glossary	99
	Programs and Services Offered	103

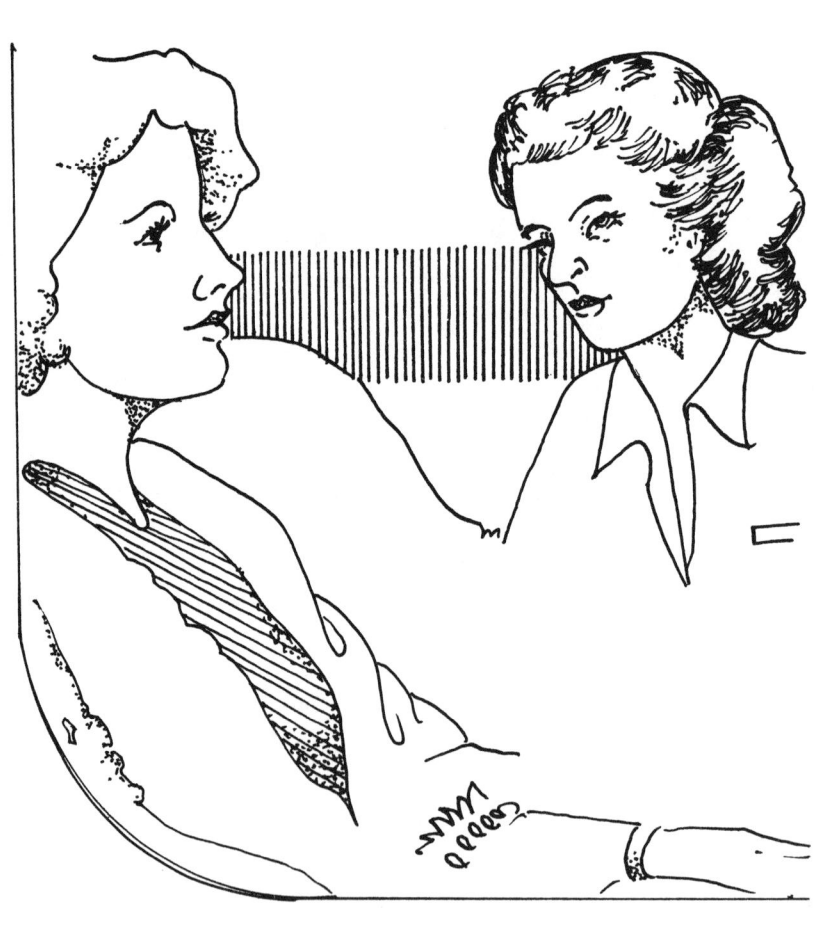

1
General Considerations

WHERE DO WE STAND IN THE 1990'S?

THE National Cancer Institute reports that by far, the vast majority of calls to its special hotline concern breast cancer. This supports my own long-held theory that women dread this condition more than any other malignancy and unfortunately, there's good reason for this fear . . .

- Breast cancer strikes 10% of the American female population
- Breast cancer is the leading cause of death of women between the ages of 40 and 44
- In 1988, there were an estimated 135,000 new cases of breast cancer in the U.S. and an estimated 42,500 deaths were attributed to it.

Yet, despite these alarming statistics, if it is "caught" early, while still small and has not yet spread, cancer of the breast is a very curable disease. In fact, it is estimated that at least 90% could be cured by early detection.

Who Is At Risk?

Which women in particular will become afflicted may depend on risk factors such as family history, age, parity, and probably many other influences about which we are not yet aware. I have devoted further discussion to this in Chapter 11, "Risk Factors".

How Can It Be Detected?

A cancerous mass may actually be present for years before it can be felt. However, we can now detect a breast cancer much earlier by using mammography (x-rays of the breast). For this reason, physicians, as well as The American Cancer Society, The National Cancer Institute, and many other related organizations, are strongly advocating mass screening of the public. Such a program would save countless thousands of lives, as well as alleviate the tremendous amount of related pain and suffering. However, until such a program is instated, the current American Cancer Society recommendations urge women to:

1. Examine their breasts one week after menstruation each month.
2. Have a physician examine their breasts at three-year intervals between the ages of 20 and 40 and annually thereafter.
3. Schedule their first breast x-ray (a baseline mammography) between ages 35 and 40 followed by annual or biannual mammograms from age 40 to 49, and annual mammograms every year after age 50.

How Is It Treated?

There have been enormous advances in the treatment of breast cancer. Women no longer must undergo the radical surgery they had to endure only a few years ago. Not only are lesser surgeries now performed, there are also a variety of alternatives which may be even better suited to the patient's particular needs.

Some of the more recent modalities (methods of treatment such as surgery, radiation therapy, chemotherapy, hormonal therapy, etc.) hold great promise. These include immunotherapy, with its development of monoclonal antibodies which attack only the tumor cells, as well as newer and better chemotherapeutic agents.

Because I feel that monoclonal antibodies may revolutionize the entire field of cancer treatment, I want to spend just a moment on them. These antibodies attack and kill cancer cells and are created naturally by our immune system. A revolutionary advancement was made when it was discovered that they could be reproduced in large numbers in the laboratory, and then injected back into the patient. The possibilities for development in this area are enormous and the promise is so extraordinary that I firmly believe that monoclonal antibodies may signal the dawn of a new era in cancer treatment.

Great strides also have been made in reconstructive surgery and women no longer need fear permanent disfigurement. In addition, thousands of patients continue to participate in studies to establish the optimum multimodalities for the best treatments.

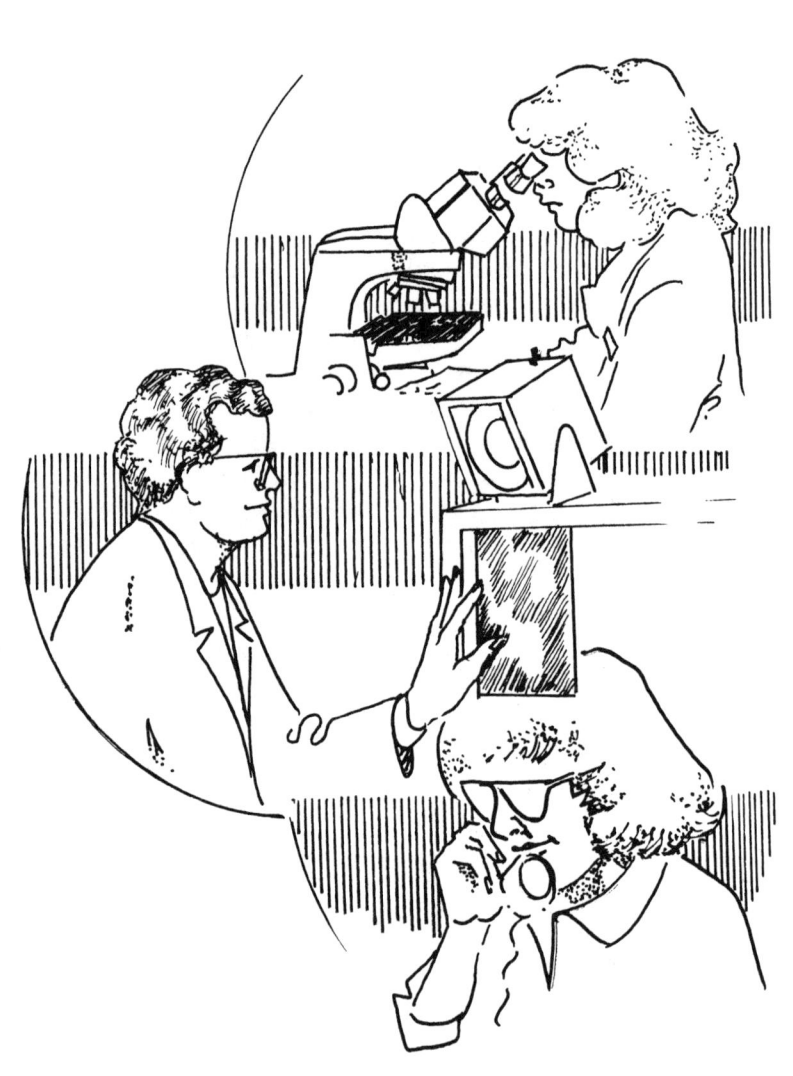

2
The Treatment Team

MOST of us have been going to a family doctor since we were very young. There were checkups, and mostly minor afflictions such as cuts, bruises, colds, allergies, and various pains. There was usually a short wait at the doctor's office, then a shot or prescription and it was all over. There was never any particular difficulty understanding the problem and how to take care of it. Occasionally, a major occurrence would surface, such as acute appendicitis. If the appendix was inflamed, the surgeon cut it out and the patient was cured and was never again bothered by an inflamed appendix.

Cancer is unlike any other disease a person will experience. By virtue of its enormous complexities, treatment requires very specific background from several diagnostic and therapeutic medical and surgical specialists. Knowledge of cancer diagnosis and therapy is expanding rapidly and this coupled with the years of required training in each specialty means that no one doctor is qualified to care for every aspect of a cancer case. As a result, a team approach has been developed. This effort, called a Multidisciplinary Approach, involves several specialists. However, by its very nature it is bound to leave the patient bewildered and feeling like a ping-pong ball being bounced around from one doctor to another. It usually leaves her feeling that, while everyone is explaining something about a particular aspect of the diagnosis and treatment, the entire picture is very difficult to grasp.

The process usually begins either when she goes to see her family doctor after finding a painless lump in her breast or when she, or her doctor, orders a screening mammogram and cancer of the breast is found.

Let's start with the first instance. When one cancer cell starts to divide and multiply, it is, of course, not palpable (able to be felt). Taking the doubling time into account, some authorities feel that as many as eight years may pass before the tumor can be diagnosed by palpation. In other words, it might have been present for years before being felt. (The usual size of a cancer when first palpated is about two centimeters or about one inch.) It is critical to understand that as the tumor grows, so do the chances that it will invade adjacent structures and spread to other parts of the body. This means that finding and removing it in the early stages will most likely effect a cure. However, if allowed to grow, simultaneously increasing its chances of spreading to other parts of the body, the odds of a cure decrease until, at some point, what began as a very treatable condition has become a fatal disease.

The solution, then, is obvious: you "catch" breast cancer early, when the likelihood of successfully treating it is highest. At present, the only means we have of detecting it before it is palpable is through a screening mammogram. The mammogram offers the distinct advantage of enabling the cancer to be "seen" before it can be felt.

The Surgeon

After finding the lump and seeing her family doctor, the patient will usually be sent to a surgeon. At this point, I would like to give you a brief overview as to how surgical procedures have advanced over the years. Just a short time ago, when mammography was still in its developmental stages, only palpable tumors were discernible so a biopsy was automatically performed. If cancer was diagnosed, the standard procedure was a radical mastectomy which was a highly disfiguring and debilitating operation. The breast and chest muscles, as well as all of the axillary (the armpit) contents were removed. This often resulted in a large, hollow area on the affected side and the arm might swell to twice its normal size. It's no wonder that some women feared the surgery more than the disease.

At that time, there was no reconstructive surgery. Once the mastectomy was completed, so was the treatment. As this was the only alternative, there were a great number of failures resulting in local recurrence in the chest wall, and spreading to other organs in the body. Radiation therapy was added to the treatment process when it was determined that it could prevent local recurrences although it did not help in overall survival rates.

The development of the modified radical mastectomy was one of the major milestones in cancer treatment. Soon after its advent, a study was completed with a group of patients who had undergone this therapy. In this experimental group, the chest wall muscles had been left intact. Compared to the control group, the cosmetic results were much better and the survival rate remained unchanged. This study has resulted in an even less complicated surgical procedure in conjunction with radiation therapy. (Lesser surgical procedures, such as a lumpectomy and radiation therapy will be discussed later on.)

So what began as a purely surgical treatment is now a team approach with the mainstay consisting of surgery, radiation therapy and chemotherapy. The actual role of these modalities, and the best combination of treatments for the various stages of cancer, is still being defined. It is clear, however, that with earlier detection and with the multimodality team approach, more people are being cured; and of those not cured, more are living longer and increasingly productive lives.

The Radiation Oncologist

Most likely, the next member of the treatment team to work with the patient will be the radiation oncologist. He or she is a doctor specializing in treating cancer with radiation (most commonly "ionizing" radiation which includes x-rays, radium, irradiation and other radioactive substances). Like every other phase of treatment, it has seen tremendous advances over the years. The first machines that delivered it were quite crude, and due to the quality of radiation, could emit only a small dose without causing severe skin burns. However, with the development of newer and better equipment (i.e. the cobalt machine and linear acceleration), combined with the experience of thousands of patients, the optimum treatment schedules and dosages are now defined and in use.

While radiation does kill cancer cells, it primarily prevents their division and, if cells cannot divide and multiply, they will eventually die. These treatments are painless and last only a few minutes. Depending on the particular type of cancer, its location and its stage, the total course of treatments can last up to five or six weeks. In some cases, radiation therapy is applied to the breast before surgery to shrink the cancer and make it operable. In others, it may be given afterwards to prevent recurrence. Years later, it can also be administered to the chest wall if there is a reappearance of the malignancy in that area.

Radiation therapy is also used if the cancer has spread (metastasized) to a bone and if the region is painful; or it that particular bone is weak and there is a chance it may break.

Possible side effects vary. Some patients may develop a dry, hacking cough which will disappear shortly after the treatments are stopped. Towards the end, the skin may become red, similar to a sunburn, but this should also pass in about two weeks. While patients undergo treatment, they are encouraged to lead as normal a life as possible.

The Medical Oncologist

Another doctor on the treatment team may well be the medical oncologist, a specialist in treating cancer by the use of one or a combination of drugs (chemotherapy). The development of multiple drug therapy was also a giant step forward in the management of malignant diseases.

This application got its start about 40 years ago when it was discovered that nitrogen mustard (then used for possible warfare application) had the potential of killing cancer cells. There have been tremendous advances and refinements since then and there are now over 75 drugs in use and several more being developed. Second-generation drugs are also available. These have the same, or more, cancer-killing effects as their predecessors and fewer side effects.

Today, a patient undergoing chemotherapy may be receiving anywhere from one to five drugs at the same time. There are two principles behind this: first, a lower amount of any one drug can be given, thus lessening side effects; second, each drug may strengthen the overall treatment by killing the cancer cells in a different manner.

Unfortunately, the regular cells that normally divide most rapidly are also affected. These are usually in the bone marrow and in the lining of our gastrointestinal tract (mouth, esophagus, stomach, etc.). This killing and damaging of normal cells gives rise to a myriad of symptoms as well as limiting how much of a drug a particular individual can take. Side effects include sores in the mouth, nausea, vomiting, diarrhea, weakness, hair loss, and many more depending on the particular agent used. For example, adriamycin is toxic to the heart, so the heart function is closely monitored and, at the first sign that it is starting to fail, the drug is discontinued.

The use of adjuvant chemotherapy, as it is called, is somewhat recent and we can continue to expect ongoing refinements and improvements with better cure and survival rates. Understandably, the newer drugs aim to be more selective in killing only the cancer cells. In 1975, The National Surgical Adjuvant Breast Project reported a landmark study in which patients had undergone a radical mastectomy followed by adjuvant chemotherapy using L-phenylalanine mustard (L-PAM). This study showed a significantly lower failure rate in pre-menopausal women receiving L-PAM as compared with studies in which only radical mastectomies were performed.

The Surgical Pathologist

A very crucial member of the treatment team is the surgical pathologist. The surgeon may have a certain impression as to whether a growth is malignant, and the radiologist may also have a definite idea. However, it is not until the tumor, or a part of it, is removed and examined under the microscope by a surgical pathologist that a diagnosis can be confirmed. Usually, in the case of a lump or thickening of the breast, an operation is scheduled to have it removed. If the abnormal area had been initially discovered by mammography, the patient is first delivered to the x-ray department. Here, guided by x-rays, a fine wire with a hook at the end is placed at the suspicious area. In the operating room, the surgeon follows the wire to the designated tissue which is removed and immediately sent to the laboratory. It is then quick-frozen, sliced into very thin sections, studied under the microscope and the findings reported directly back to surgery. If it is benign, the surgeon can stop at this point or if malignant, continue with the definitive operation as predetermined between the patient and her doctor.

After surgery, the specimen is returned to the pathologist for further study to ascertain the extent of the disease. He or she will report on the size of the primary tumor, the margin of normal tissue safely present around it, the appearance of the tumor cells and the lymph nodes; and whether the lymph nodes are positive (contain tumor cells) or negative (free of tumor cells). A crucial factor is the closeness of the malignancy to the chest wall muscles. This information is not only vital for prognostic value, but it may determine, in part or completely, both therapy and rate of cure.

There are now a number of important decisions to be made, one being whether or not the patient should have chemotherapy. The conclusions may hang in the balance until the pathologists's final report is obtained and a conclusive diagnosis is made (one or two days).

The surgical pathologist will also examine suspicious tissues for possible recurrence. For example, let's say that a few months after surgery, the patient and her doctor feel a small lump in the armpit (axilla). The doctor thinks it is probably just scar tissue, but to be certain, removes it by a local excision. The tissue is then sent to the surgical pathologist who reports back as to its nature. If necessary, appropriate therapy can then follow.

The Diagnostic Radiologist

The diagnostic radiologist is a physician who uses any of a number of imaging devices to determine the extent of the primary disease. These methods include x-rays, ultrasound, radioactive materials, angiography and CAT scans.

For example, the diagnostic radiologist may detect a small non-palpable tumor through routine mammography or perhaps a find lung cancer in a chest x-ray ordered to evaluate a cough. The discovery of a primary malignancy such as a lung or a breast cancer will then launch an extensive exploration to determine its extent. This may include a CAT scan of the abdomen to inspect the liver and a bone scan to rule out cancer to the bones. Other organ systems (i.e. the heart, lungs, and kidneys) may also be analyzed to assess if the patient is well enough to undergo the designated therapy.

After therapy is complete, follow-ups will be made to ensure that the tumor has not recurred—their form and frequency determined by the type and extent of cancer. If it is to return, it will most likely do so in the first five years after it was initially found and treated.

The Oncology Nurse

Specializing in the care of the cancer patient, the oncology nurse is a special breed. I have worked with them for several years, and have found that the very nature of their vocation attracts kind and caring people. Oncology nurses must possess an exceptional virtue of understanding and empathy with their patients and their patients' families. As he or she will see the patient daily, a very close relationship will usually develop.

The Radiation Therapy Technician

The radiation therapy technician is the person who performs the daily radiation treatments and like the oncology nurse, must be proficient and technical as well as understanding and sympathetic. While the patient undergoes treatment, the technician will be in close communication with her family, and will subsequently develop a close and reassuring relationship with everyone involved.

Emotional Counselors

Cancer affects not only the afflicted person but the entire family as well. The diagnosis of a mother with breast cancer is one of the most traumatic events that a family will ever experience yet responses of different members will vary. It is safe to say, however, that everyone, including the patient, will undergo various and highly emotional reactions as time goes on. As these include fear, desperation, anger, loneliness and a sense of hopelessness, the assistance of a professional counselor can be highly beneficial during this period.

Such a person, a psychiatrist or psychologist, or perhaps a member of the clergy, is specifically trained to aid in alleviating much of this anxiety and can treat both the patient and her family members. This person will help each individual to see that his or her feelings are both understandable and natural, and, that with compassion and open communication, their associated distress can be eased.

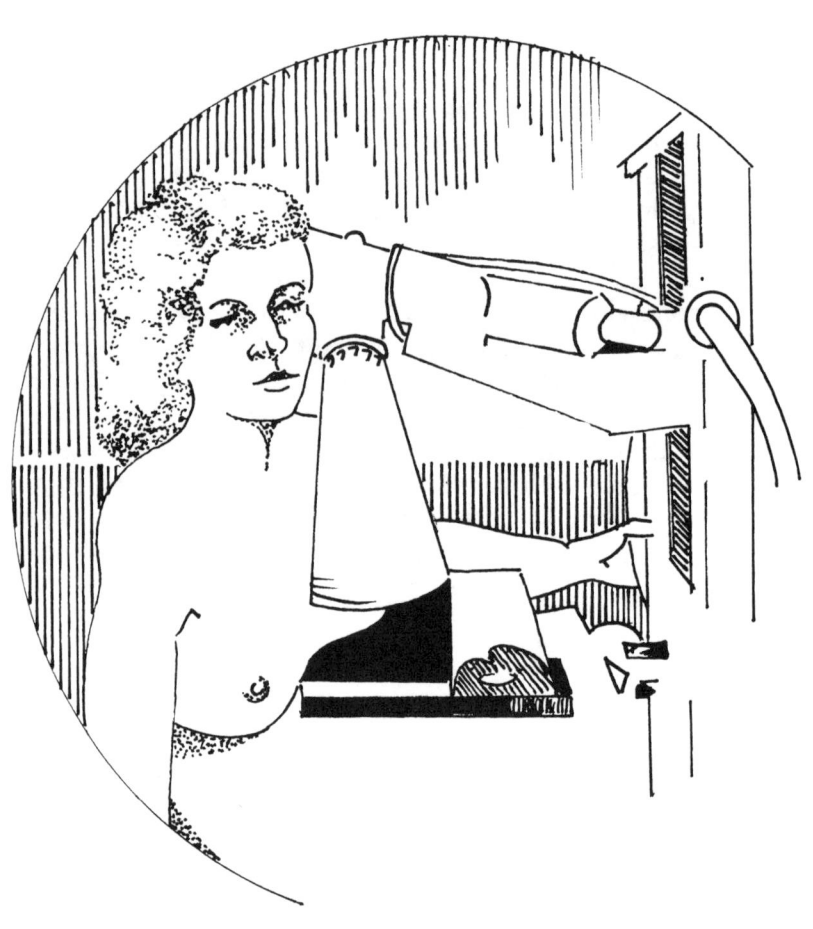

3
Diagnosis of Cancer of the Breast

EVERY woman should examine her breasts once a month. By doing so regularly, she will come to know her particular breasts and therefore, can detect any change.

For most women, there are probably few occasions more distressing and alarming than finding that growth. This fear is quite understandable since breast cancer is so prevalent and most people know someone, or of someone, who has had the disease. In addition, many women have heard horror stories of mutilating surgery and radiation burns as well as the sickness and debilitation brought on by chemotherapy.

Clinical Diagnosis

There is obviously cause for concern and the discovery of any lump or thickening must be checked immediately (as I will say over and over—early detection is the key to cure and survival).

In almost three out of four cases, the doctor does not discover the growth. Instead, the woman brings it to her physician's attention and this is why such a tremendous effort is made by the medical community to increase public awareness of breast self-examination (BSE). While about 80% of all such masses are benign, there is no way to differentiate by feel between a benign growth and one that is malignant. A woman's breasts undergo continual changes and such occurrences as menstruation, age, pregnancy, menopause, or even a blow to the breast can cause changes that may be confused with a tumor. (I once had a patient with a hard lump in her breast that I felt certain was malignant. Upon its removal, the surgical pathologist informed me that it had been caused by an inflammatory mass around a thorn. The patient was a gardener, had gotten too close to one of her plants and a thorn stuck in her breast.)

While breast cancer can occur at any age, it is rare below the age of 30 (less than 1%). The peak incidence is between 45 and 55. The age group between 40 and 60 comprises 50%; but overall, the 35 to 70 segment will include about 85% of women afflicted.

A very common finding in a young woman with a non-tender breast mass is a benign fibroadenoma, which is simply a benign tumor. Fibroadenoma mostly occurs between the ages of 20 and 40, and is usually indistinguishable from cancer until it is removed. Since the possibility of malignancy is present at any age, the lump should be excised. And, early diagnosis is the key to cure and survival.

Mammography

The major concern in all malignancies is the rate at which cancer cells multiply. We begin with the premise that one cell from either the duct system or the mammary glandular tissue goes awry and becomes a cancer cell which then multiplies and becomes two, the two become four, the four become eight, etc. So, if we can estimate the time it takes for this doubling, we can guess how long the tumor has been there. (It is felt that with the use of mammography, cancer may be detected up to eight years before it can be palpated.)

Since survival and cure are directly related to early diagnosis, the problem is obvious—how can we "see" the tumor before it can be felt? This is where mammography comes into play. While it has been around for some time, only over the last 10 to 15 years has its technology become advanced enough to provide reliable and accurate information. Today's x-ray machines and related equipment emit a very low dosage of x-ray while giving the radiologist optimum pictures.

A radiologist looks for two basic things in a mammogram: microcalcifications and/or the tumor itself. These microcalcifications appear as little white spots on the x-rays and resemble grains of salt. In the very early stages, this may be all one can see and can be a very fortunate finding since the removal of a minute grouping of, let's say, a few millimeters, may result in cure rates of well over 95%. If the tumor is in a stage called "in situ" which is microscopic, and still contained, the cure rates will be 100% after a simple mastectomy. The presence of an actual tumor implies a more advanced state of the disease and the radiologist then observes its shape. Those which are round or oval with sharp margins are more likely to be benign than those that are irregular and have spiked margins.

There are other types of calcifications which are benign and of no consequence. They may have resulted from old trauma or infections; and in older patients or diabetics, we sometimes see calcification of the arteries in the breast.

Biopsy

If the tumor is palpable, the biopsy is no problem. The surgeon either removes it or excises a wedge and sends it to the surgical pathologist. The surgical pathologist usually does a "frozen" section and calls the surgeon with a diagnosis within minutes.

On the other hand, since a growth discovered through mammography can be virtually impossible for the surgeon to find, a procedure has been devised enabling the radiologist to localize it. This takes place in the x-ray department. First the tumor, or area of microcalcification, is seen in two views, and the radiologist places a needle containing a wire at the site of the abnormality. A second set of films is then taken to ascertain if the tip of the needle is close to the spot. If it is either in the tumor, or very close, the needle is withdrawn and the wire left in place. Now, the patient is sent to the operating room where the surgeon follows the wire and removes the tissue at its tip. X-rays are again taken, this time to be certain that the correct area was removed. If it was, the specimen then goes to the surgical pathologist who proceeds with a "frozen section" and calls the surgeon with the diagnosis.

A decision can now be made whether to proceed with the definitive surgery. Prior to the procedure, the surgeon and patient will have discussed the possibility of finding a malignancy, and may have elected to wait and discuss the treatment options afterwards as it is generally agreed that a few days between biopsy and surgery are not harmful. Some prefer to have "everything" done at the same time, while others wish to learn the exact diagnosis before consenting to any type of treatment. Both are acceptable and the surgeon should respect the patient's previously expressed desires.

Staging

A cancer spreads when small clumps of cells from the primary site (where it first develops) break off and travel through the bloodstream or the lymph nodes to another location where they multiply and grow. Therefore, anytime it is detected, a great deal of effort is made to determine both its local extension and to ascertain if it is now in the bones or organs. Each of the over 100 kinds of cancer has its own characteristics, one being how it extends locally as well as its pattern of spread at a distance. For example, while breast cancers can travel to any part of the body, they have a tendency to expand to the bones, liver, lungs and brain.

There are three good reasons for the meticulous search that is conducted to ascertain spread. First, treatment will vary with the breadth of the disease. Second, a prognosis will be made based on the extent of cancer in other organs. Finally, it will determine the patient's "staging" which is a judgement of which of several stages (categories) her illness should fit. Using this classification, her doctors can establish the most effective therapy by evaluating the efficiency of current treatment among those with the same degree of disease. The factors comprising each stage have been agreed upon by physicians throughout the world (they will be covered later on in this section). This is called Uniform Staging, and while all types of cancer are staged, not all have been done so by universal accord, as has breast cancer.

For example, as there is international agreement that Stage I cancer of the breast is defined as a malignancy of two centimeters (about one inch) or less in the greatest dimension, treatments for Stage I from all over the globe can be compared. Also, new therapies that fail to do well can be discarded. Staging also enables progress to continue in the war against cancer as it ensures continuous communication between doctors throughout the world.

Generally speaking, a patient is staged in two manners. The first is clinical staging. This concerns the amount of cancer the doctor thinks is present before the pathologist examines the surgical specimens. For example, the doctor might palpate what seems to be a 1.5 centimeter breast mass with no spread to the axilla. After surgery, the pathologist finds that the cancer was actually three centimeters and that it has spread to the 10 to 25 lymph nodes examined. This would not be an unusual case. When the pathologist examines the breast tissue and the contents of the axilla, which is negative about one third of the time, he or she will find microscopic cancer that the physician could not feel. Now, the patient is restaged. In our example, this particular patient went from a clinical Stage I with negative nodes, to a pathological Stage II with positive nodes. All else being equal, this difference means that the cancer was more advanced than initially thought, and it may determine as to whether the patient is treated with chemotherapy.

There are three factors in staging breast cancer. First is the size of the primary tumor of the breast. Depending on its size, these are classified TIS, T1, T2, T3, or T4.

TIS or "tumor in situ" as it is called, deserves special mention. It is adjacent to those cells where it originates, has not invaded contiguous structures and when found and treated, is considered 100% curable. The tumor is so small that it cannot be felt either by the patient or the doctor and is located only by mammography (which may show only a few small calcifications).

To illustrate, most cancer of the breast originates in the duct systems that channel the milk to the nipple. If the cancer is in situ and originates from there, it will be confined to that system. Once it penetrates to the outer structure, it is considered invasive and of a more serious nature because it has access to the blood vessels and lymphatic system by which it can spread. The next step is to determine if the tumor has invaded the adjacent lymph nodes. These are part of the lymphatic system which drains fluid from the tissue and replaces it into the circulating blood through a series of ducts. These small, bean-shaped structures act as a filter to stop and destroy any foreign substance such as bacteria or cancer cells. When they are negative for cancer cells, it means the cancer is most likely still localized in the breast. This, of course, indicates a better prognosis.

The earlier the disease is found, the less chance of it having spread. When the lymph nodes are positive, the cancer is no longer localized and cancer cells are probably circulating in the blood. This means a worse prognosis and more extensive therapy.

The extent of the involvement of the lymph nodes is

critical. Cancerous lymph nodes which are not able to be felt before surgery, but are detected by the pathologist through the microscope, are certainly less ominous and easier to control than the large matted nodes easily felt by both the doctor and the patient. Thus, lymph nodes are also classified as to the extent of involvement. These are N0 (meaning no tumor involvement), N1, N2, or N3.

The last item to consider in staging is whether the cancer has extended and is now growing in one or more other areas. As noted before, the usual organs of spread for breast cancer are the bones, liver, lungs and brain. This is noted as M0 or M1. M0 means no known distant spread, and M1 means there is known distant spread of the cancer.

Putting it all together, then, the staging of breast cancer is as follows:

AMERICAN JOINT COMMITTEE ON STAGING OF CANCER OF THE BREAST

PRIMARY TUMOR (T)

TIS: In Situ
T1: Tumor two centimeters (about one inch) or less in greatest dimension
T2: Tumor more than two centimeters but not more than five centimeters in greatest dimension
T3: Tumor more than five centimeters in dimension
T4: Tumor of any size with direct extension to the chest wall or skin
    T4a: Fixation to the chest wall
    T4b: Edema (swelling), ulceration of breast skin, or satellite skin nodules confined to same breast
    T4c: Both of the above
    T4d: Inflammatory carcinoma (a specific kind of breast cancer that is very malignant)

Nodal Involvement (N)

    N0: No palpable axillary lymph nodes
    N1: Movable axillary lymph nodes

N2: Axillary nodes containing growth and fixed to one another or to other structures
N3: Supraclavicular (above collar bone), or Infraclavicular (below collar bone) nodes containing growth or edema of the arm

Distant Metastasis (Spread)

M0: No known distant metastasis
m1: Distant Metastasis

It should be noted that this staging system has been somewhat simplified for our purposes.

Tumor Type and Histology

Following the diagnosis of the initial frozen section, the pathologist examines the entire surgical specimen and makes permanent slides of the tumor and lymph nodes. The study which deals with these minute structures of tissue is called Histology.

The histology of the tumor relates directly to the overall outcome of the disease. Well-developed and mature-looking tumor cells tend to be slower growing and less malignant than those which are poorly and immaturely developed. Two other probable indications of a worse prognosis are microscopic spread of the tumor to the lymphatic system and blood vessels; and whether the border of the tumor is smooth and round, or irregular with jagged edges that appear to be piercing and infiltrating the nearby tissues. Those with a smooth border, of course, carry a better prognosis.

Hormone Receptor Assays

Your doctor will order a hormone receptor assay which involves excising a piece of the tumor and than assaying (testing) it for the presence or absence of hormone receptors. These structures on the cell's surface allow it to bind and use specific hormones, including estrogen and progesterone, for therapeutic purposes.

Tumors are classified as estrogen receptor (ER) positive and ER-negative, or progesterone receptor (PR) positive and PR-negative. About two thirds of all women with breast cancer are ER-Positive. ER-Positive women are more likely to respond to hormone therapy and have a better overall prognosis, independent of other factors, such as lymph node status, size of the primary tumor and age, than ER-negative women. They also experience a longer disease-free period after primary therapy, and show a greater overall survival on the average.

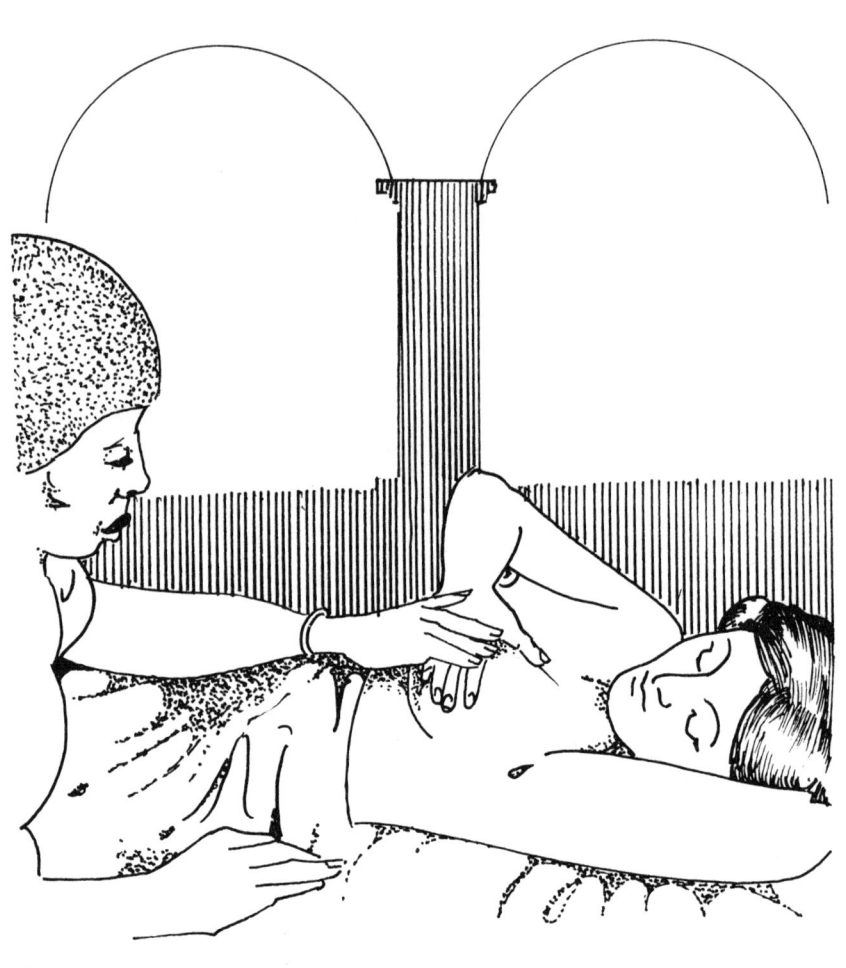

4
Treatment of "Early" Breast Cancer

THERE are a number of processes which have led to dramatic changes in the treatment of breast cancer over the last 10 to 15 years:

1. A deeper understanding of the various biological processes involved.
2. Major advances in the technology for earlier detection.
3. Tremendous progress in chemotherapeutic drugs and the knowledge of how to use them.
4. The enormous potential in the field of immunotherapy, still in its infancy.

With current public awareness and the knowledge of the importance of early diagnostic capabilities of mammography, 80% of breast cancers when first treated, are considered "early"—Stage I or Stage II. In this chapter, we will discuss only the treatment of the Stage I and Stage II disease.

As physicians, when we stage a patient, we consider three primary factors. The first is the size of the primary tumor in the breast—the smaller the better, of course. Next we determine if there has been spread to the axillary lymph nodes. Those which are larger, matted, and confluent (growing into one another) carry a worse prognosis than the smaller and single node. Finally, we consider whether there has been spread to other parts of the body (metastasis).

The smallest-sized tumor that we can detect and treat is called "in situ". These are confined to the area where they originate, are uniformly non-palpable and can be identified only by mammography. When these cancers are found and treated they carry a 100% cure. Next in order of prognosis are Stage I cancer (less than two centimeters in size). The more advanced stage would be a tumor two centimeters or less but involving the lymph nodes in the axilla. In Stage II, the tumor is over two centimeters but less than five. If there are positive axillary lymph nodes (contain cancer) the prognosis is worse than if they are negative.

The Treatment

The treatment of breast cancer began in the late 1800's with the introduction of the radical mastectomy by Dr. William Halstead. During the ensuing period, women usually had advanced disease by the time they sought medical treatment and the mastectomy was an extensive and mutilating operation. It left the patient disfigured and sometimes with severe physical impairments. Believe it or not, this was still the procedure of choice in the early 70's.

Today, although surgery continues to be the primary therapy, this particular form has nearly been abandoned. The treatment is evolving and will probably continue to do so for years. There are scores of studies, involving thousands of patients, to determine the best means and ironically, one of the major problems in cancer research is that it may not recur for up to thirty years (though the average length of time is three years). This means that obtaining meaningful data from a new therapy may take a tremendous amount of time.

It was initially assumed that cancer spread from the breast to the lymph nodes and then, at some point, from there to the rest of the body. However, current thinking is that it travels in both the bloodstream and the lymphatic system; and can spread throughout the body very early in its development. The importance of the immune system in ridding the body of cancer, and also in preventing its spread, is now being unraveled and recognized. Since, in Stages I and II, the cancer is considered to be limited to the breast and perhaps the lymph nodes, it is possible to remove and rid the body of all the cancer. This can be accomplished through surgery and/or radiation therapy. If the lymph nodes contain cancer, the probability of it invading other organs is very high. Further treatment, which includes radiation, drugs, hormones or immunotherapeutic agents may, be warranted.

The Mastectomy

The modified radical mastectomy and the total mastectomy are the most common surgical procedures for Stages I and II breast cancer. In each operation, the entire breast is removed and the major chest muscles left intact. The difference is that, in the modified radical mastectomy, some or most of the axillary lymph nodes are removed. In a total mastectomy, most or all are left intact. These methods are superior to the old radical mastectomy since chest wall muscles are preserved, the arm regains strength and there is no hollow area beneath the collar bone. Also, reconstruction is easier, and there is usually no swelling of the arm. The results of these lesser procedures are about the same as the more mutilating and disfiguring radical mastectomy.

Other Surgical Procedures

The next treatments can be characterized as more limited surgical procedures. They are the quadrantectomy; partial mastectomy; and a local excision sometimes called a lumpectomy and are used in conjunction with radiation therapy.

The quadrantectomy removes that quarter of the breast containing the tumor, along with the overlying skin, the sheath covering the chest wall muscles, and sometimes, the axillary lymph nodes.

A partial mastectomy, also known as a segmental mastectomy, removes the tumor, a two to three centimeter wedge of normal tissue surrounding it, and a portion of the overlying skin and underlying membranes that envelop the breast and chest muscles.

Local excision, also called lumpectomy or tylectomy, removes just the tumor, or the tumor and a small margin of surrounding tissue. The skin and membranes are left intact. While in some cases, most of the axillary lymph nodes are removed, the general rule is to take only a few to obtain a sample for microscopic examination for tumor cells. Up to 40% of the time, positive axillary lymph nodes (containing cancer cells) had been considered clinically negative (not containing cancer cells) by palpation. Therefore, the axillary node sampling is very important to help stage the patient and determine the treatment course.

Limited surgical procedures are usually followed by radiation therapy to the affected breast, the chest wall and the axilla. This normally starts within a week to ten days after the surgical procedure.

Followup

The first visit to the radiation department will take up to an hour and in some cases, may be an intimidating experience. This need not be the case, as the patient usually finds that radiation therapy personnel will be very friendly and reassuring.

The initial treatment is longer as the radiotherapist must take an x-ray to ascertain the accuracy of the fields where the patient is to be treated. From here on out, however, the setup time may be ten to fifteen minutes, and the actual radiation therapy only about two or three minutes per field. The patient will then undergo about five weeks of treatments, usually daily, excepting weekends, for a total of 5000 rads (one rad is the basic unit of radiation dose).

Toward the end, the treated area will resemble a bad sunburn but this usually subsides about two weeks following the completion. Patients normally continue their daily routine while on treatments and some report no side effects whatsoever. Others say that they don't quite have the same energy level as before but these symptoms also subside with the termination of treatment. There may be some changes in the breast itself. It may feel firmer, and the overlying skin may have increased or decreased sensations. A very few patients may develop a temporary dry hacking cough and some shortness of breath. This is caused by radiation to the lung within the chest.

A week or two after the end of the therapy, the patient starts her second phase (or booster dose). This is done with either a radioactive implant or by the use of an electron beam. To the patient, there is little difference in the electron beam therapy and the previous treatment. She will go to the radiation therapy department daily for an additional five to ten days. With radioactive material implantation, she is usually hospitalized for three days.

The implant procedure is generally conducted under local anesthesia. The first step is to place plastic tubes through the breast tissue. Once in place, they are filled with seeds of a radioactive material called irridium which deliver an approximate dosage of 2000 rads. The implant remains in place for fifty to sixty hours after which the tubes are simply pulled out and the patient is sent home.

There are numerous ongoing patient studies to establish the best forms of therapy for Stages I and II and although total mastectomy, with the axillary dissection, remains standard, there is increasing enthusiasm for some lesser surgical procedures plus radiation. In fact, the results have been so encouraging that this could very well become the normal treatment for Stage I and Stage II in the future.

The benefits of a minor surgical procedure compared to the total mastectomy and axillary dissection are obvious. First of all, any necessary reconstruction is not as complicated or extensive and the results are superior. Even more important are the continued advances in chemotherapy and immunotherapy. Since 25% of those in Stage I will develop a recurrence, the current trend of a more systemic approach (chemotherapy and immunotherapy) is likely to continue and improve.

Not all patients are good candidates for a limited surgical procedure, though, and one major factor is how strongly a woman feels about the preservation of her breast. Of further significance is the size of the malignancy. A tumor over four centimeters or one which is large in relation to the size of the breast might contraindicate a lesser procedure. Patients with pendulous (hanging) breasts may not be considered because they do not tolerate the radiation therapy as well.

This is a very personal decision, and the pros and cons of any particular form of therapy should be fully explained to the patient by the treating physician.

Chemotherapy

The word "chemotherapy" refers to the use of drugs that kill cancer cells throughout the body. They are taken by mouth or by injection, depending on the particular drug. When the treatments are given in conjunction with surgery or radiation therapy, it is called adjuvant chemotherapy.

Once confined to advanced and metastatic disease, chemotherapy is now frequently used as adjuvant therapy to the primary surgery and/or radiation treatments and routinely follows when the lymph nodes are involved (Stage II). In addition, further therapy must be considered for those women in the 25% recurrence segment of Stage I.

Lately, the goal has been to identify those patients who are at high risk (carrying a worse prognosis than others of similar stage) and to treat them with further chemotherapy and/or hormonal therapy. Determinants of who would fall in this category include the histological grade of the tumor, the presence or absence of hormone receptors, and the number and size of the positive lymph nodes in the axilla. The larger the positive lymph nodes and the more that become confluent with each other, the worse the prognosis.

On one hand, we know that cancer deposits are left behind in high risk patients. On the other, even with our excellent technology, there can easily be microscopic deposits that are undetectable. To provide an idea of the magnitude of the problem, a deposit on the head of a pin would probably contain about one million cancer cells, and a deposit the size of a pea would contain about a billion. It is obvious that while the amount might be enormous, the task of finding these deposits is extraordinarily difficult. Therefore, while surgery and radiation therapy will contain the primary cancer and its local spread to axillary lymph nodes, systemic therapy (chemotherapy, hormonal therapy and immunotherapy) is employed to control the small deposits that have already traveled to one or more organs and cannot be seen or detected with our current technology.

Adjuvant chemotherapy for breast cancer began in 1958, with the study of a drug called thio-TEPA then being administered for two days following surgery. The improved survival rates of the women receiving thio-TEPA prompted numerous other clinical studies. While the final outcome as to the optimum treatment will not be known for many years, there are highly encouraging preliminary findings indicating that adjuvant chemotherapy prolongs the disease-free interval and can lengthen overall survival in certain patients. The benefits among node-positive pre-menopausal women have been the most striking.

There are currently several chemotherapeutic drugs which attack the cancer cells at different stages during reproduction. Cancer cells develop and multiply much more rapidly than healthy cells and are therefore more susceptible to damage by chemotherapeutic drugs. Also, because of the affects of various drugs on different steps in the cell cycle, they are more potent when used in combination. It is not unusual for a patient to be treated by three to five drugs simultaneously, as no single combination has proven superior to date. This use of multiple drugs is called combination chemotherapy. (Several of those currently in use, as well as particular combinations, are addressed in the chapter on Chemotherapeutic Agents).

Unfortunately, no chemotherapeutic drug treats only cancer cells and the healthy cells that divide most rapidly are also affected. Included are those in the lining of the gastrointestinal tract, the bone marrow (which produces the white cells in our blood), and the hair follicles. One drug is particularly toxic to the heart. Side effects depend on particular combinations and also on the patient's general health (people who are unwell and bed-ridden will obviously not do as well as those in relatively good shape).

Specific symptoms relate to whichever organ system is affected (ulcers of the mouth, nausea, vomiting, bleeding and diarrhea) because of the involvement of the gastrointestinal tract (since the cells in its lining divide very rapidly, the killing effect of the chemotherapeutic drug quickly affects them and their sloughing off gives rise to the side effects). In addition, the decrease in white cell production results in a greater susceptibility to infection and also produces general fatigue, nervousness, and general irritability. These symptoms disappear when the treatments are discontinued.

Adjuvant Hormone Therapy

Because certain breast cancers depend on the ovarian (female) hormones for their growth, removal of the ovaries will cause some of these malignancies to shrink.

With this in mind, physicians utilize a variety of means to manipulate the hormones to the patient's benefit.

The various approaches include either surgical removal or radiation of the ovaries, surgical removal of the adrenal glands, and even surgical removal of the pituitary gland. In some cases, the administering of male and/or female hormones also seems to be beneficial although the exact mechanism as to how this works is unclear.

Two recent advances have helped refine and develop the use of hormone therapy. First, the development of a laboratory test enabling the physician to determine who will respond to the treatment. This is called an estrogen receptor assay and involves the examination of a piece of the cancer for the presence or absence of estrogen receptors. If the tissue has estrogen receptors, the patient is called ER-Positive. If there are no estrogen receptors, she is referred to as ER-Negative. About two-thirds of women with breast cancer are ER-positive and approximately 60% will respond to hormonal therapy. ER-negative women seldom respond to the treatment. A further refinement is to test for progesterone receptors. If a woman has both estrogen and progesterone receptors, her chances of responding to hormonal therapy is up to 80%.

The second step in the advancement of hormone therapy was the introduction of drugs which work as effectively as surgery or irradiation to inactivate the hormone-producing glands.

A powerful anti-estrogen drug now being studied is called tamoxifen. Demonstrating a remarkable lack of toxicity and side effects, tamoxifen is not only excellent for the treatment of advanced cancer, it also has applications in early stages. ER-positive patients with either positive or negative lymph nodes have responded well to treatment and several clinical studies combining it with chemotherapy also show encouraging results. Unfortunately, the drug usually does not seem to help those pre-menopausal women who are ER-Negative.

Side effects of hormonal therapy are well-tolerated. While those taking a drug called Magase have reported weight gain, such an increase may be perceived as a benefit rather than an unwanted complication since advanced breast cancer is frequently associated with weight loss. Breakthrough vaginal bleeding and hot flashes are other possible results.

Summary of Treatment for Early Breast Cancer

In Situ and/or Minimal Breast Cancer

Tumor small and confined to the area where it originates. Not palpable. The five year survival is greater than 95%.

1. Quadrantectomy, partial or segmental mastectomy with or without axillary lymph node sampling.
2. Excisional biopsy or lumpectomy with radiation therapy with or without simultaneous axillary lymph node sampling.
3. Total mastectomy with or without axillary lymph node sampling.

Stage I

Tumor two centimeters or less and negative lymph nodes. The five year survival is 85%.

1. Quadrantectomy, partial or segmental mastectomy with axillary node dissection and radiation therapy.
2. Excisional biopsy or lumpectomy with separate axillary node dissection and radiation therapy.
3. Modified radical or total mastectomy with axillary dissection.

Adjuvant Therapy

1. For ER-Negative Patients:
   Adjuvant chemotherapy with a proved effective regimen.

2. For ER-Positive Patients:
   Adjuvant tamoxifen with an established schedule.
3. Under clinical evaluation are other adjuvant chemotherapy and/or hormonal therapies.

Stage II

Tumor between two and five centimeters or positive axillary lymph nodes. The five year survival is 66%.

1. For tumors less than four centimeters in size and adequate tumor free margins:
   A. Quadrantectomy, partial or segmental mastectomy with axillary node dissection and radiation therapy.
   B. Excisional biopsy or lumpectomy with a separate axillary node dissection and radiation therapy.
2. For any Stage II:
   A. Modified radical or total mastectomy.
   B. Radical mastectomy in certain selected circumstances if needed to accomplish complete tumor resection.

Adjuvant Chemohormonal Therapy

1. For pre-menopausal women with positive axillary lymph nodes—adjuvant chemotherapy with a proved effective regimen. Treatment usually not to exceed one year.
2. For post-menopausal women with positive axillary lymph nodes—adjuvant tamoxifen therapy with a regular established schedule.
3. In axillary lymph node negative women:
   A. For ER-Negative Patients:
      Adjuvant chemotherapy with a proved effective regimen.
   B. For ER-Positive Patients:
      Adjuvant tamoxifen with a regular established regimen.
4. Under clinical evaluation are protocols evaluating new types of chemotherapy and/or hormonal therapy.

While I have provided a general outline and framework of the treatment of early breast cancer, the actual therapy given any particular patient may vary a little—or a lot. To involve every factor (including the general health and age of the patient), and every possible treatment plan would be beyond the scope of this book. The recommended procedure may have to be modified because of, let's say, preexisting kidney or heart disease that would limit the type and kind of chemotherapy or surgery. Since every patient is unique, she and her physician must ultimately determine her particular course. This also holds true for advanced and recurrent breast cancer.

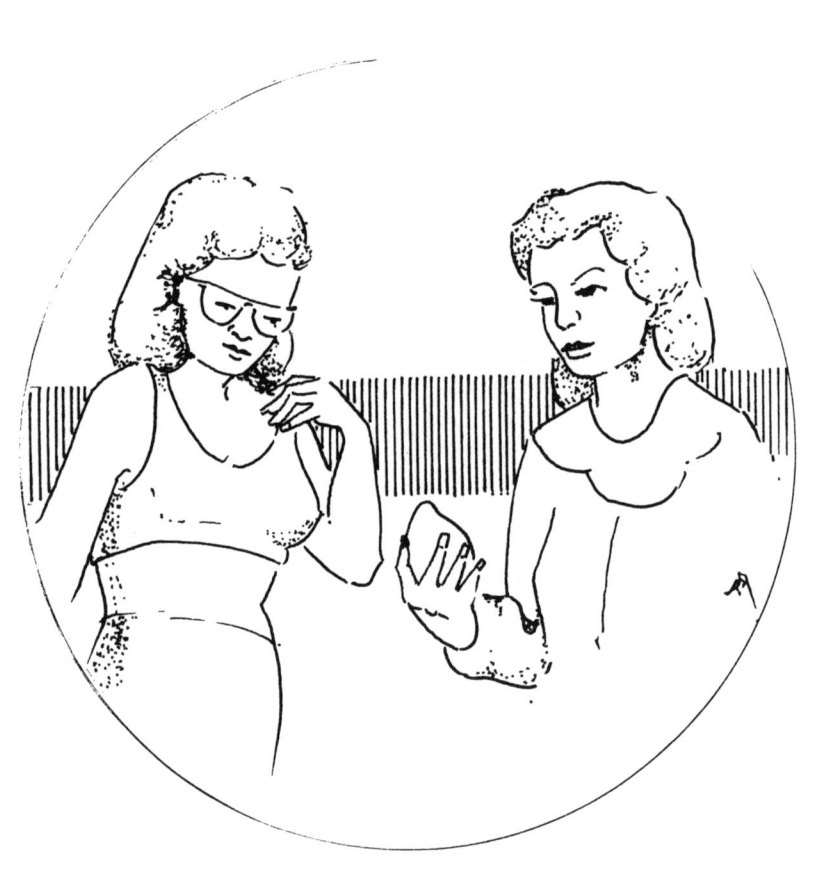

5
Treatment of Advanced Breast Cancer

ADVANCED cancer of the breast can be divided into three categories: Stage III, Stage IV and Recurrent Cancer. Fortunately, due to increased public awareness and more refined diagnostic techniques, there are fewer Stages III & IV malignancies and today, about 80% of breast cancers, when first diagnosed, can be classified as "early".

Stage III is confined to the breast and/or the local lymph nodes. It can be further divided into IIIA and IIIB which is a very important distinction from a treatment standpoint. Stage IIIA consists of a primary breast tumor of more than five centimeters in greatest diameter and/or axillary lymph nodes considered to have tumor growth and also fixed to one another or to other structures. This stage is considered operable.

In Stage IIIB, the primary tumor is invading the underlying chest wall muscles and/or cancerous lymph nodes extend to above or below the collar bone and may be so far-reaching that they are causing swelling of the arm.

In the advanced stages, a mastectomy is often not the first choice of treatment as the cancer may have progressed too far into other organs for it to have any effect. For Stage III, radiation therapy is important in the control of the local disease and chemotherapy is recommended for the small pockets that may be present in other sites but are virtually undetectable. If there has been a good response to the radiation therapy and/or the chemotherapy, the patient may then be evaluated for a mastectomy.

Stage IV cancer has traveled to other organ systems. Common sites of spread are the lungs, liver, bone, and brain and the prognosis is poor. In up to 20% of the patients, there is a good response to treatment with long term remission (stablization or reversal of the disease) although long disease-free survival to the extent compatible with cure is rare. Surgery is usually limited to a biopsy establishing the diagnosis and determining the estrogen/progesterone receptor status. Radiation to the breast and lymph nodes and sometimes a mastectomy, is used to control the local disease. Radiation therapy also plays a major role in the palliation (easing) of symptoms, especially those caused by spread of this cancer to bones (bony metastasis).

Summary of Treatment for Stage IIIA Breast Cancer

1. One of the following surgical procedures for initial treatment:
    A. Modified radical mastectomy
    B. Radical mastectomy
2. Because of the high risk of local recurrence for this stage, radiation therapy should be considered as part of the overall treatment plan:
    A. Pre-operative radiation therapy
    B. Post-operative radiation therapy
3. Chemotherapy regimens with or without hormones are given in conjunction with the above surgical procedures. Some of the effective combination chemotherapy regimens commonly used are:

CMF: Cyclophosphamide + methotrexate + fluorouracil

CMAF:	Cyclophosphamide + methotrexate + doxorubicin + fluorouracil
DMFP:	Cyclophosphamide + methotrexate + fluorouracil + prednisone
CMFVP:	Cyclophosphamide + methotrexate + fluorouracil + vincristine + prednisone
L-PAM & F-FU:	Melphalan + fluorouracil (for menopausal women)
L-PAM, 5-FU & Tamoxifen:	Melphalan + fluorouracil + tamoxifen (for post-menopausal women whose tumors are estrogen/progesterone positive)
CA:	Cyclophosphamide + doxorubicin

Summary of Treatment for Stage IIIB Breast Cancer

1. Surgery is usually limited to a biopsy for diagnosis and to obtain tissue for a receptor assay. This is followed by radiation therapy to the affected breast and regional nodes. If the response is good, this may be followed by a cone-down field and further irradiation plus radiation implants to the tumor-bearing area. If the response is poor, a mastectomy may be performed, if technically feasible; or continued radiotherapy with a cone-down field.
2. After the surgery and radiotherapy described above are complete, one of the following chemotherapy regimens may be considered:

CMF:	Cyclophosphamide + methotrexate + fluorouracil
CAF:	Cyclophosphamide + doxorubicin + fluorouracil
CMFP:	Cyclophosphamide + methotrexate + fluorouracil + prednisone
CMFVP:	Cyclophosphamide + methotrexate + fluorouracil + vincristine + prednisone
CA:	Cyclophosphamide + doxorubicin

3. If combination chemotherapy is contraindicated, one of the following hormonal therapies may be recommended for patients whose tumors are positive for estrogen and progesterone receptors after the surgery and radiotherapy described above are complete:
   A. Surgical removal of the ovaries (oophorectomy) for pre-menopausal patients.
   B. Tamoxifen for post-menopausal patients.
   C. Estrogen for post-menopausal patients.
   D. Progesterone therapy.
   E. Androgen (male hormones) therapy for pre-menopausal or post-menopausal patients.
4. Under clinical evaluation are:
   A. Studies utilizing combination chemotherapy initially followed by surgery and/or radiation therapy, and maintenance chemotherapy.
   B. Chemotherapy using newly developed chemotherapeutic agents or biologicals (interferon, etc.) for patients whose local disease is not controllable by standard measures.

Summary of Treatment for Stage IV Breast Cancer

1. A surgical biopsy to establish the diagnosis and estrogen/progesterone receptor levels. Radiation therapy or a hygenic mastectomy may be recommended to control local disease.
2. If liver, lung, and brain disease are absent and estrogen and progesterone receptor status is positive, hormonal therapy is an excellent first treatment. One of the following equivalent approaches can be used:
   A. Tamoxifen or surgical removal of ovaries (oophorectomy) for pre-menopausal patients.
   B. Anti-estrogen therapy with tamoxifen for post-menopausal patients.

C. Estrogen therapy for post-menopausal patients.

D. Progestational agents for post-menopausal patients.

3. If lung, liver or brain disease is present, or estrogen and progesterone receptor status is negative, one of the following combination chemotherapy regimens will produce equivalent results:

CMF: Cyclophosphamide + methotrexate + fluorouracil

CAF: Cyclophosphamide + doxorubicin + fluorouracil

CMFP: Cyclophosphamide + methotrexate + fluorouracil + prednisone

CMFVP: Cyclophosphamide + methotrexate + fluorouracil + vincristine + prednisone

CA: Cyclophosphamide + doxorubicin

4. Under clinical investigation are numerous protocols that call for evaluating the role of various hormonal and combination chemotherapy and also newly developed chemotherapeutic agents and biologicals such as interferon.

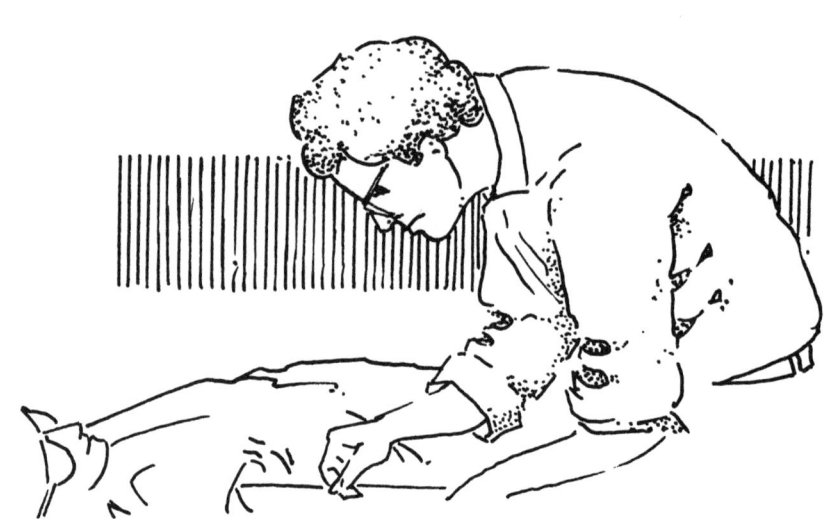

6
Recurrent Cancer of the Breast

IN order to increase the chances of containing recurrent breast cancer, it is crucial to "catch" it at the earliest possible time. Due to its high probability of reappearance, patients are watched closely after their initial treatment and are usually examined every three months for the first two years, every six months for the next three years, then annually. Although most recurrences will appear within three years for Stage I and two years for Stage II, breast cancer can return as many as thirty years later so patients must be followed throughout their lives.

When a recurrence is encountered, appropriate laboratory and x-ray diagnostic procedures are undertaken much as if it were newly discovered because as before, the extent of the disease determines the therapy to be employed as well as the prognosis.

A recurrence may be localized such as in the chest wall or axillary lymph nodes; however it may also appear at some distant site, i.e. the lungs. Symptoms of lung involvement (pulmonary metastasis) are usually a persistent cough or hoarseness. Metastasis of the liver may give rise to such symptoms as nausea, loss of appetite, jaundice and liver enlargement. Headaches, convulsions or abrupt changes in behavior may indicate brain metastasis. The first sign of bone involvement is often a tenderness over the affected area.

Summary of Treatment for Recurrent Breast Cancer

1. If the recurrence is limited to bone, lymph nodes and skin, and the estrogen/progesterone receptor status is positive or unknown, and the disease-free interval exceeds two years:
    A. Tamoxifen or surgical removal of ovaries (oophorectomy) for pre-menopausal patients, or radiation castration, if surgery cannot be performed.
    B. Anti-estrogen therapy with tamoxifen for post-menopausal patients.
    C. Estrogen therapy for post-menopausal patients.
    D. Progesterone therapy for post-menopausal patients.
2. If there is local recurrence only to skin and local lymph nodes, treatment options would be surgery and/or radiotherapy.
3. Patients who respond to hormonal therapy, and then relapse should be considered for other forms of hormonal therapy such as:
    A. Those previously utilized therapies in (1) above, or
    B. Androgen therapy (male hormones) for pre-menopausal and post-menopausal patients.
4. If lung and/or liver and brain disease is present, and estrogen and progesterone receptor status is negative, or if the disease-free interval is less than two years:

   A-CMF: Cyclophosphamide + methotrexate + fluorouracil
   B-CAF: Cyclophosphamide + doxorubicin + fluorouracil
   C-CMFP: Cyclophosphamide + methotrexate + fluorouracil + prednisone
   D-CMFVP: Cyclophosphamide + methotrexate + fluorouracil + vincristine + prednisone

E-L-PAM: Melphalan (for frail, debiliated patients)
F-CA: Cyclophosphamide + doxorubicin
5. Under clinical investigation are several protocols involving different hormonal, combination chemotherapy, and newly developed chemotherapeutic agents and biologicals such as interferon.

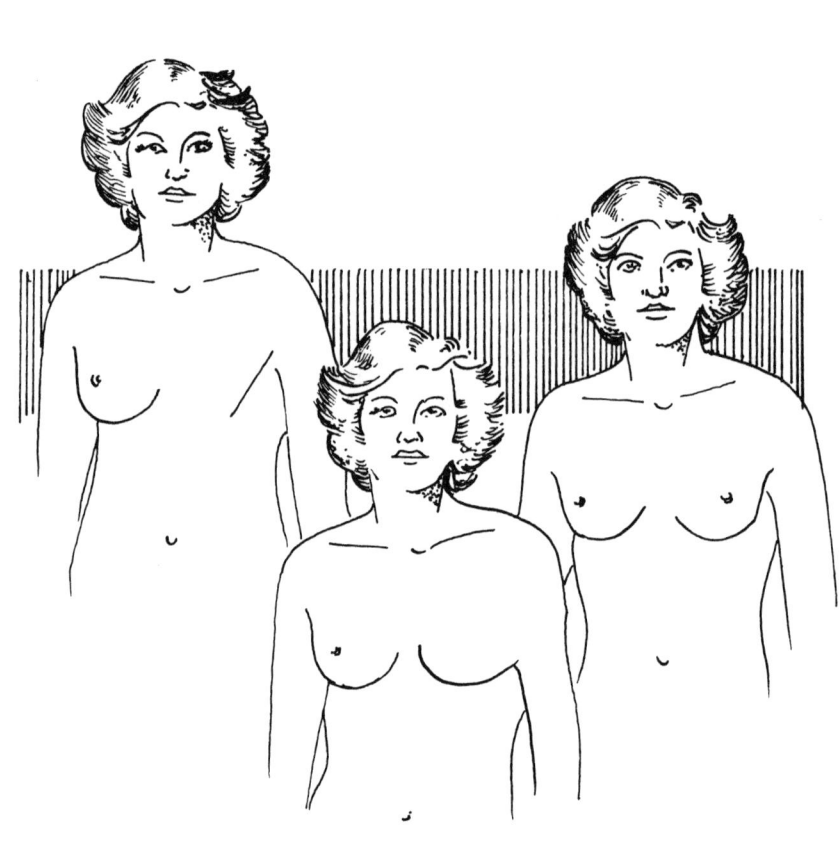

7
Breast Reconstruction

WHILE there are still a surprising number of people who are unaware that breast reconstruction is available and now state-of-the art, it is becoming an increasingly popular elective for several reasons . . .

- The modified radical mastectomy and lumpectomy have all but replaced the radical mastectomy, thereby greatly simplifying the reconstruction procedure.
- Modern technology has resulted in the development of silicone gel implants which have the feel of normal breast tissue. Generally a sac made of silicone rubber, and filled with silicone gel, the implant is available in all sizes and shapes. (This procedure is not to be confused with the liquid silicone injections once used for breast enlargement. Those produced a number of complications and were eventually banned by the Food and Drug Administration.)
- The development of a technique of tissue transfer from one site to another for grafting. This is an important advancement on which to elaborate:

A common site of tissue transfer is from the back and called the Latissimus Dorsi Reconstruction (incidentally, pioneered and developed by an old friend and medical school classmate, Dr. John Bostwick, a plastic surgeon). In this procedure, skin, fat, and the latissimus dorsi muscle (a broad, flat back muscle located below the shoulder blade) along with its blood supply, are transferred to the front by tunneling the flap of tissue under the skin to the front of the chest. This method is used when the mastectomy surgery has left too little skin and muscle for a simpler procedure. An implant is then placed related to the new chest muscle. As time goes by, other back muscles compensate for the loss of the latissimus dorsi muscle and there is very little disability.

Another common tissue transfer procedure is the Abdominal Advancement Reconstruction—often used for large-breasted women. Skin and fat is removed from the chest and abdomen, below the mastectomy site, and advanced to the breast area.

Another technique also used for women who have had a great deal of skin and muscle removed is the Rectus Abdominus Reconstruction. The rectus abdomini are two parallel muscles in the abdomen. The surgeon cuts one of them and then tunnels this flap of skin, fat, and muscle, along with its blood supply, to the appropriate area in the shape and contour of the other breast. Transferring tissue from the abdomen has the added benefit of tightening the stomach, the so-called "tummy tuck".

The Simple Implant is used when the chest wall muscles are intact and there is enough good skin to cover the implant. A small incision is usually made through the mastectomy scar, and the implant is placed either under or over the chest wall muscles. This sometimes takes place as out-patient surgery.

The next method, Tissue Expansion, is used when the quality of the skin is good, but the quantity is not sufficient to allow implant placement. A tissue expander is placed under the skin and muscle and then filled with a sterile fluid. Weekly, over the next two or three months, the physician will inject increasing amounts of fluid to enlarge the expander and stretch the tissue over it. When the tissue has reached the desired expansion, the device is removed and a permanent implant put into place.

The decision as to when to begin reconstructive procedures varies from surgeon to surgeon. Some prefer the time of the initial surgery while most wish the tissues to be well healed, usually three to six months later. It is generally advisable to wait until chemotherapy and/or radiation therapy has been completed.

While some women are satisfied with the results at this point, others go on to have their nipple reconstructed. Because breast tissue is attached to them and may be harboring cancer cells, the nipple and areola are always removed during the total or modified mastectomy. There is usually a waiting period of up to several months after the initial reconstruction in order to allow the breast to settle into its permanent shape. At this point, minor surgery can reshape and better match the reconstructed breast with the other breast.

There are various ways to reconstruct the nipple and areola. Tissue from the upper inner thigh or skin from behind the ear is often used for the areola. The nipple can be formed by using tissue from the opposite nipple or creating one from the reconstructed breast itself. Another is the use of skin from the vaginal lips.

The decision to have breast reconstruction is a very personal one. Some women, not wishing to endure more surgery, want no part of it. Others feel that it will make them feel whole again and eager to resume life. In general, those who do proceed are satisfied with the results.

When contemplating reconstruction, the first step is to find a plastic surgeon in whom you have confidence and with whom you can talk freely. The physician should be frank, thorough and forthcoming about what you can realistically expect. Try to also speak with other women who have had the same experience.

ANATOMY

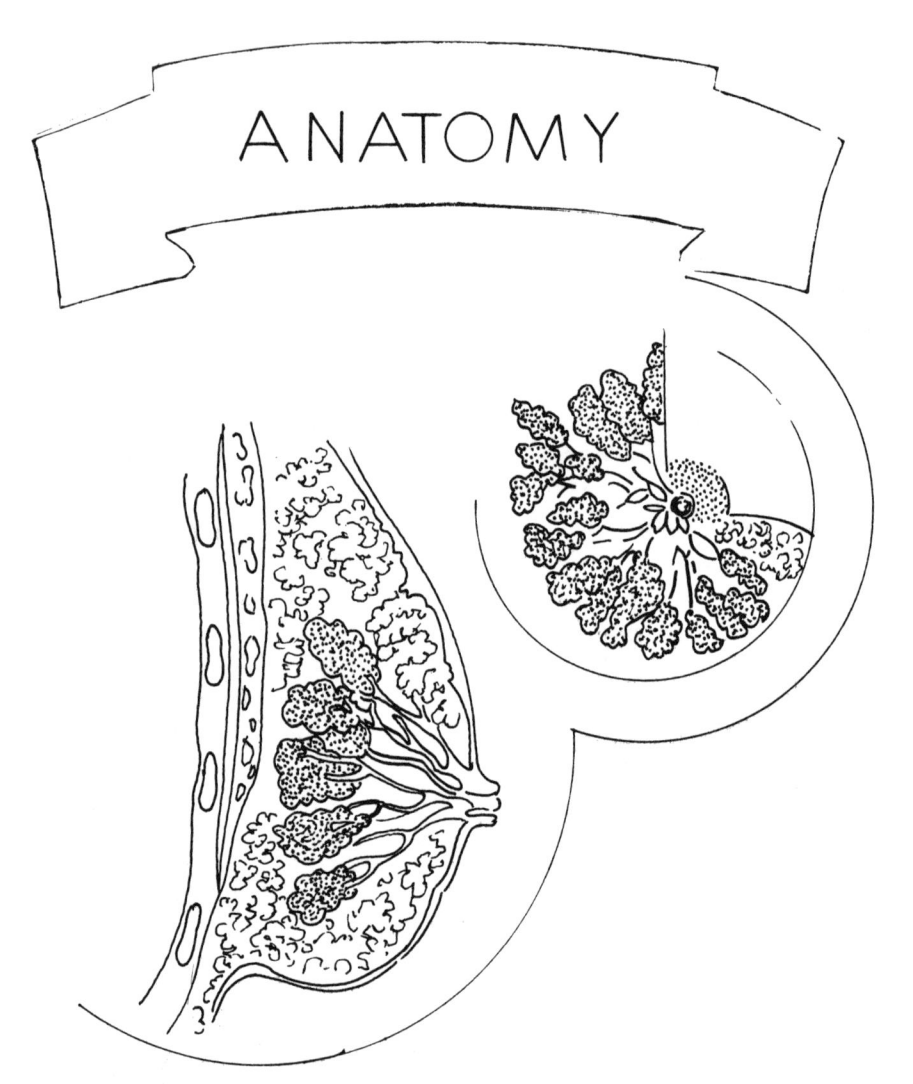

8
Anatomy

THE actual anatomy of the breast is not very complicated. It consists mainly of cells that produce milk, and a system of ducts to funnel the milk to the nipple. In addition, there are supporting structures, blood vessels and fatty tissue. The major problem for the physician is the degree of breast dissimilarity from patient to patient, and even variations in the same patient at different times of the month, etc. As breasts are naturally nodular, determining which nodule is important can be very difficult. This is why breast self-examination, mammography, and regular check-ups by a physician are highly recommended.

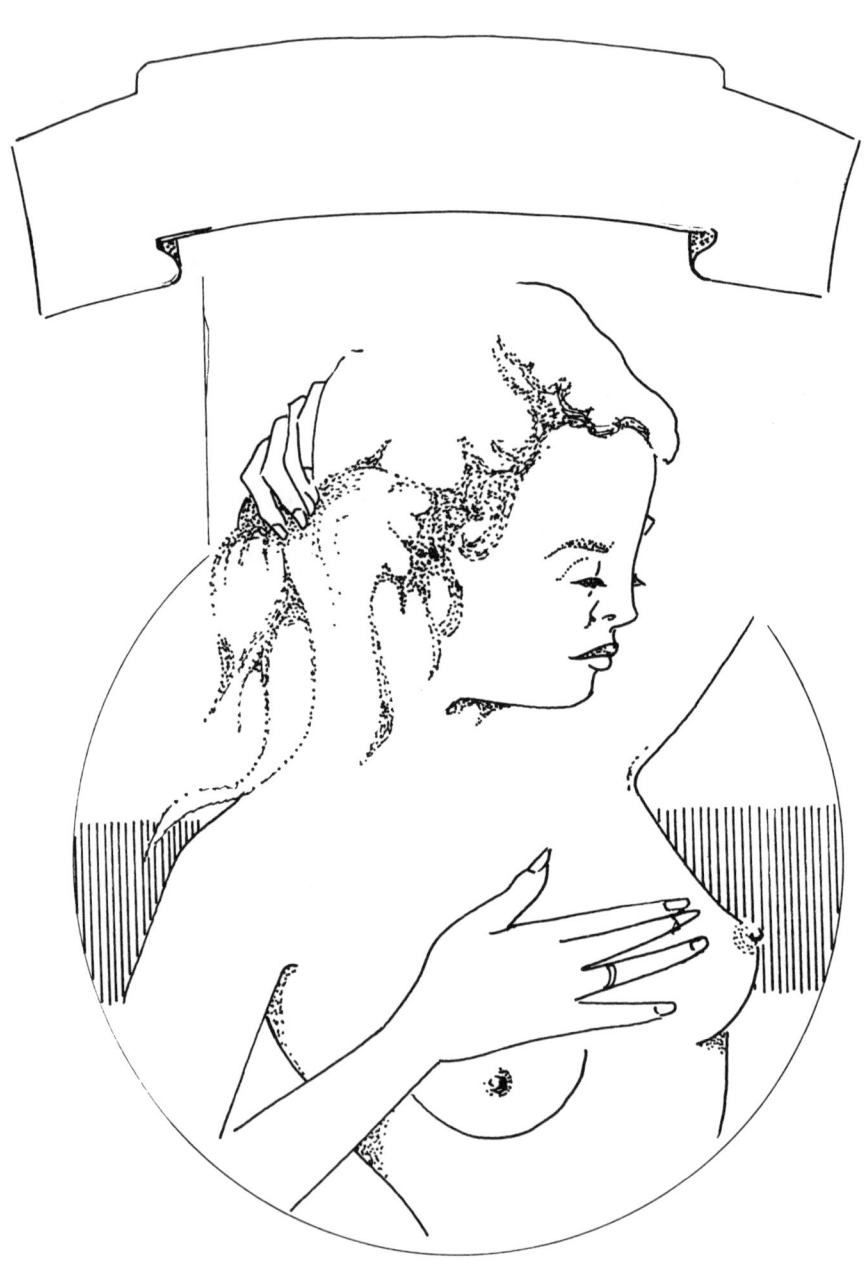

9
Breast Self-Examination

SINCE the outcome of breast cancer depends almost entirely on early discovery, it is critical to have regular mammograms. The first screening mammogram should be done between the ages of 35 and 40, followed by annual or biannual mammograms from 40 to 49, and annual mammograms every year after 50. In addition, the patient's own, very vital, responsibility, is breast self-examination (BSE). Each woman's breast is unique insofar as its size, shape, and texture are concerned, so she can best appreciate any subtle change. For this reason, BSE is strongly recommended by The American Cancer Society, The National Cancer Institute and all other interested associations and individuals.

BSE must take place monthly, preferably at the same time. If you menstruate, you should wait two or three days after your period ends so that your breasts are least likely to be swollen and tender. It should follow a step-by-step procedure, and you might consider placing a card in the bathroom or shower area as a reminder.

The question as to the extent of the advantage provided by BSE and/or mammography has been addressed extensively by The National Cancer Institute. It has released the following series of illustrations which should remove any doubt about the efficacy of BSE and mammography.

BREAST SELF-EXAMINATION (BSE)

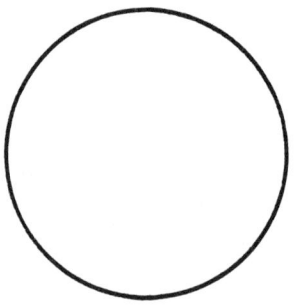

A. The average size tumor found in a woman who is untrained in BSE. Keep in mind that there are about one million cancer cells in a volume the size of a pinhead and a growth the size of a pea can contain one billion cells.

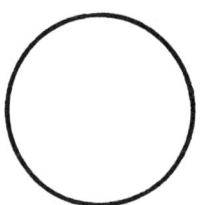

B. Average size tumor of a woman practicing regular BSE.

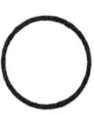

C. Average size tumor found by a woman practicing occasional BSE

D. Average size tumor found by the first mammogram.

●

E. Average size tumor found by regular mammogram.

BREAST SELF-EXAMINATION (BSE)

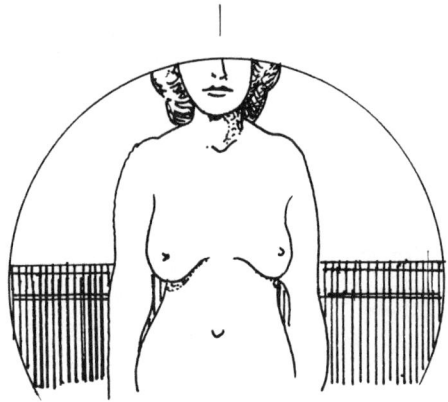

The first step is to just stand in front of the mirror and look at the breast for anything unusual, such as puckering, dimpling or scaling of the skin.

While still watching yourself in the mirror, clasp your hands behind your head and press your hands forward. Again, check for any puckering or dimpling, and especially for any asymmetry between each breast.

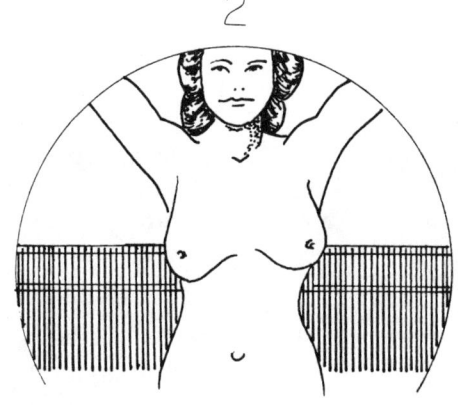

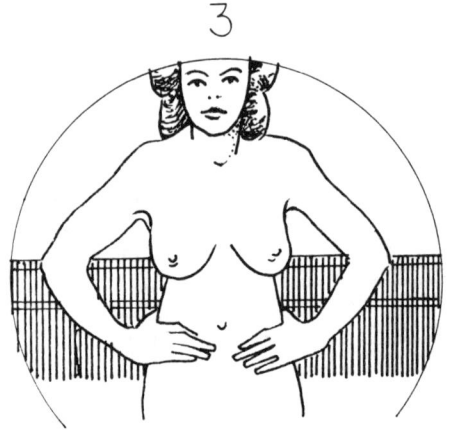

Next, place hands on your hips and press while bowing slightly toward the mirror as you pull your shoulders and elbows forward.

Now, raise one arm and with the other (using the flat part of your four fingers) feel and examine your breast. Examine in small circles, slowly moving all around the breast including the armpit and the area between the armpit and breast. Do this to both breasts.

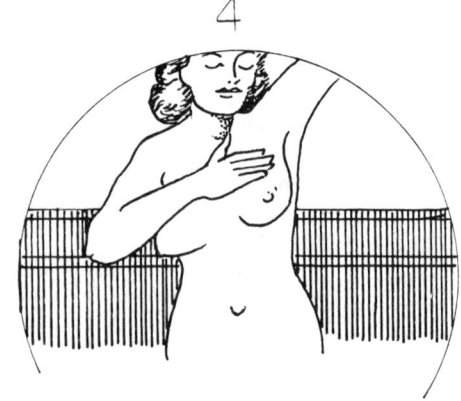

BREAST SELF-EXAMINATION (BSE)

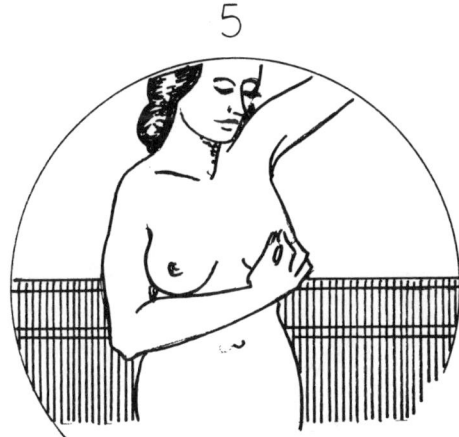

Gently squeeze the nipples for any discharge.

Repeat steps 4 and 5 while lying on your back. Placing a pillow or a towel under the shoulder of the breast you are examining will help to flatten the breast and make it easier to examine.

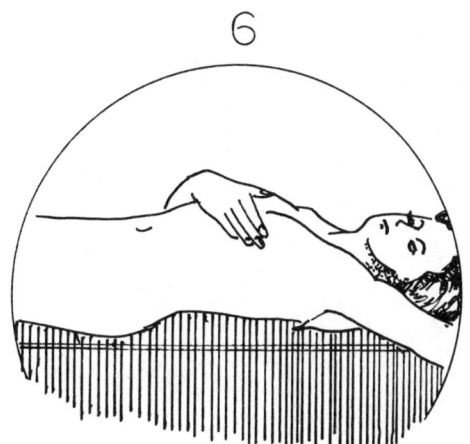

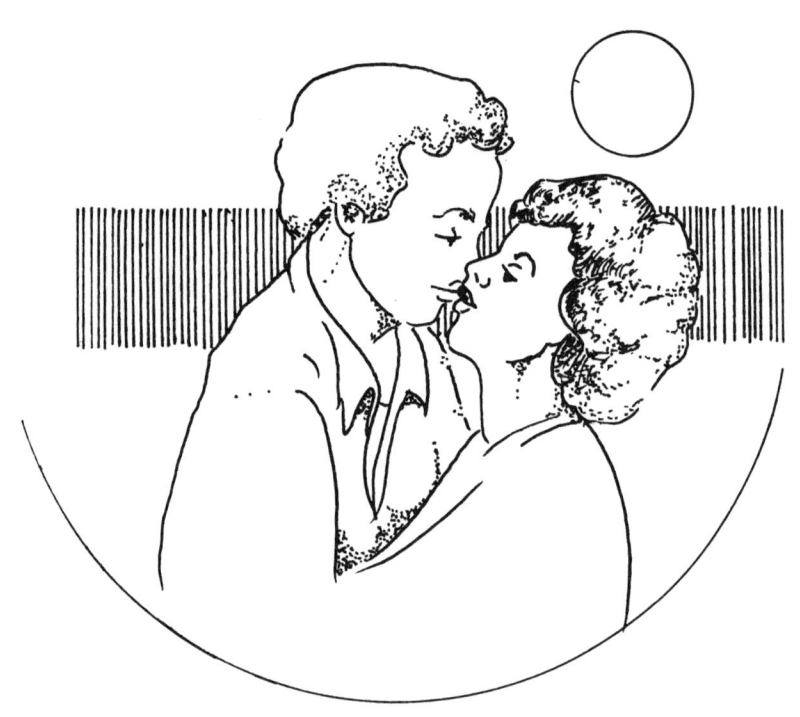

10
Sex and Breast Cancer

THE ordeal of breast cancer goes far beyond surgery, adjuvant therapies, and uncertainty of the future. There is also an emotional trauma involving the very foundation of a woman's being. She often experiences a loss of self-worth as well as her sense of femininity and may fear that her husband or lover will find her unattractive. With this in mind, it's interesting to note that statistically, patients who undergo a lesser surgery with radiation therapy, actually do better and have less recurrences. I believe that a very strong factor may be their more positive self-image: As they still have both breasts, they don't have the feelings of anxiety or loss of self-esteem that might accompany the modified radical or radical mastectomy.

During treatment, definite physical changes occur throughout the entire body. Their degree depends on the individual's general health as well as the type of therapy. For example, a patient undergoing a lumpectomy may experience only minor discomfort while a radical mastectomy normally results in weeks or months of recovery and rehabilitation.

In addition, if she is undergoing radiation or chemotherapy, she will definitely experience (in some cases, highly unpleasant) side effects.

A woman should be open and frank about the physical effects of her treatment and a husband or lover must understand that because physical sex may be uncomfortable, there is greater need for warmth, love and understanding. This is when the necessity is greatest for loving words and reassurance, warm embracing and cuddling. The process of communication and caring is, of course, on-going but is especially important during these stressful times. As treatments end and life begins to resume a more normal course after this difficult but shared experience, the relationship may develop into a stronger bond and union between these two people.

My Darling

My darling, we met—I loved you instantly.
Maybe it was what you said—or how you said it.
Maybe it was the twinkle in your eyes,
 or the smile on your face.
Maybe it was the hot pink pants,
 or the tight-fitting jeans.
Maybe it was the wiggle in your walk—
 or the "giggle in your talk".
I don't really know why I fell in love with you
 I only know I did.

Now there's a deeper love.
Now there's a love beyond that physical attraction.
A love that is deep and emotional,
A love that goes beyond reason
 and intellectual understanding.
A love that is spiritual . . .
 and all encompassing.
A love that does not depend on the physical body
 . . . but on the inner self and soul.
A love that will only grow deeper and stronger
 with each passing day . . .
And even a serious affliction cannot drive it away.

—P. R.

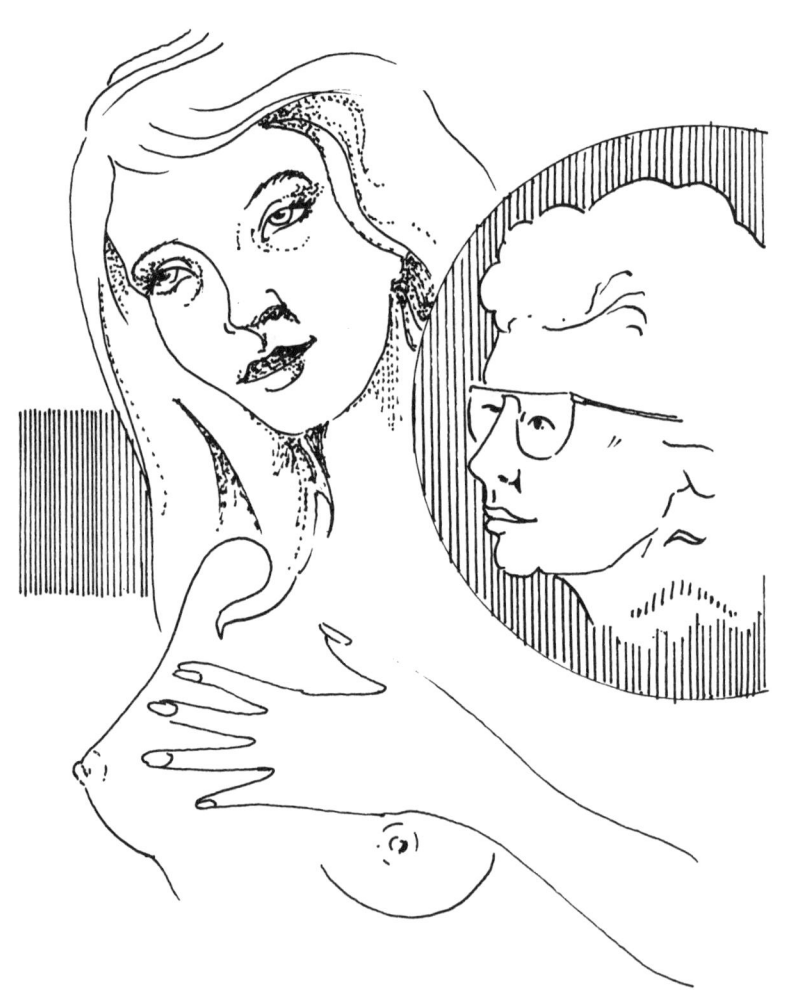

11
Risk Factors

WE all know that a certain portion of the population will develop cancer, just as a definite percentage will be involved in a car accident or will acquire coronary artery disease. Certain factors, such as drinking, will increase the risk of a car accident. Certain factors, such as sedentary existence, smoking and a diet high in saturated fats will increase the risk of a heart attack. So it is that certain factors will increase a woman's chance of developing cancer of the breast.

Although a woman may possess such characteristics, they will not necessarily lead to breast cancer. However, she should be followed more closely by her physician and must be punctual about breast self examinations and mammography.

You should note the following risk factors:

- Breast cancer will develop in one out of every 10 women.
- In 1988, there was an estimated 135,000 new cases of breast cancer and an estimated 42,500 deaths.

On a more individual basis, the following aspects of a woman's life should be considered . . .

- Family history. If family members have had the disease, she has a greater chance of developing it than a woman the same age with no such history.

- Parity. The odds of breast cancer increase relative to the age at which a woman bears her first full term child. The risk is less for woman under the age of 30 bearing their first child. There is also a greater risk in women who remain childless (nulliparous).
- Age. Cancer of the breast is rare under age 30 but the incidence increases with age. Those who menstruate earlier and those who enter menopause later have a greater risk factor.
- Benign fibrocystic breast disease. This is a clinical entity characterized by breast pain and tenderness that fluctuates with the phases of the menstrual cycle, becoming more attentuated before menstruation. Fibrocystic disease may also signify microscopic changes that are considered abnormal but not malignant. Some physicians feel that certain of these benign changes may be pre-malignant or that they share a common cause (etiology) with breast cancer.
- Previous personal history. Those who have already had a malignancy of the breast have greater odds of getting in the other than the general population.

It should be noted that while women taking birth control pills show no increased incidence, they do appear to demonstrate a higher rate of fibroadenoma (a benign tumor that occurs in young women). Since it can't be differentiated from a malignancy when discovered on x-ray or by palpation, it is removed. Research indicates that fibroadenomas found in women taking "the pill" do not differ from those in women using other methods of birth control.

A frequently-voiced concern is the relationship of radiation exposure to the development of breast cancer. When the x-ray was first developed, little was known of its potential deleterious effects. (I remember, as a youngster, looking into the fluoroscope at a local shoe store, needlessly exposing the lenses of my eyes to irradiation.) Indeed, there is no question that this is a risk factor which has been demonstrated in at least three groups of women:

1. Those treated for postpartum mastitus (inflammation of the breast after childbirth) by x-ray.
2. Those treated for tuberculosis by x-ray.
3. Those women who survived the atom bombs of Hiroshima and Nagasaki.

In each of these groups, the incidence of breast cancer was higher than in the non-exposed population. The minimum latent period was ten years. Research shows that a woman's age when she was exposed is important, with the ages of 10 to 20 showing the maximum sensitivity. It is certainly obvious why people are no longer treated for infections with x-ray.

A common question concerns potentially harmful effects of the x-ray dosage received during a mammogram. This seems to present no problem because current equipment is designed to emit a minimum dose. To my knowledge, there has never been a case where cancer was attributed to mammography, and health professionals generally agree that the benefits of these x-rays far outweigh any theoretical hazards.

While the presence of risk factors does not necessarily lead to breast cancer, neither does their absence mean that a woman is immune. In fact, there is no apparent risk factor in the vast majority of cases.

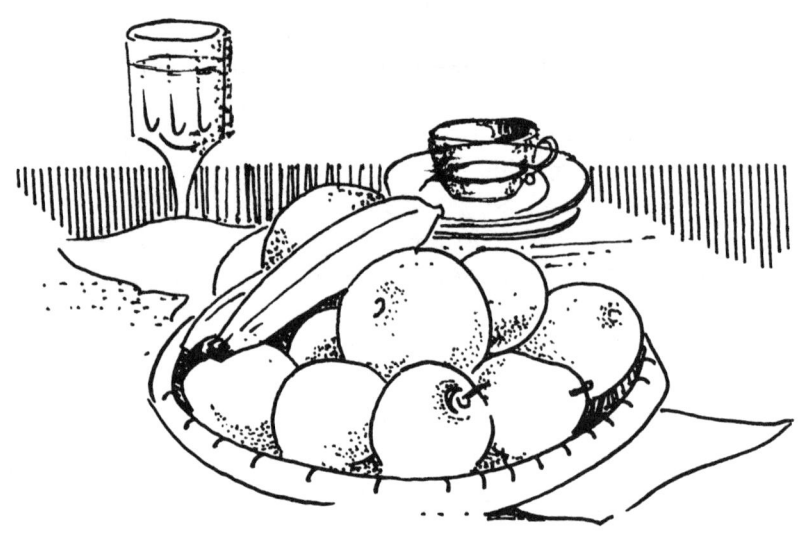

12
Cancer Prevention

ALTHOUGH this book focuses on malignancies of the breast, I feel it's important to include a chapter on cancer prevention in general. We are working on the assumption that you will be cured of your disease and are in a sense starting over and getting a new lease on life.

A great number of cancers are related to lifestyle . . . good news since that can be changed. We can now ask what went wrong in the first place and what can be done to minimize our chances of contracting it?

Current epidemiological (the study of the patterns of diseases as they affect the population) evidence suggests that 80% of all cancers diagnosed in Western society could be avoided. Dr. P. Boyle of the Analytical Epidemiology Department at the International Agency for Research on Cancer in Lyon, France, cites the following statistics regarding cancer deaths:

- 35% can be attributed to diet
- 30% can be attributed to tobacco usage
- 10% can be attributed to infection
- 4% can be attributed to occupational exposures
- 3% can be attributed to alcohol
- 2% can be attributed to pollution

1% can be attributed to medicine and medicinal procedures

−1% can be attributed to food additives

Let's review some specific changes we can make to reduce our chances of contracting cancer of any sort.

Smoking

First, if you smoke—quit! Beyond the shadow of a doubt, smoking is the single most preventable health problem and cause of death in the United States. It kills 300,000 Americans each year, 142,000 from cancer alone.

Smoking causes approximately 80% of all lung cancer and has also been implicated in cancers of the mouth, larynx, esophagus, pancreas and bladder. And cancer is only part of the health problems brought about by smoking. There are few things in life as sad as seeing a once healthy, robust person with chronic emphysema. These formerly active people have destroyed their lungs to a point where they can no longer transfer life-giving oxygen from the air into their systems. In more advanced cases, patients cannot even take a few steps without running out of breath. Smoking also causes hardening of the arteries, and is a major factor in heart disease.

Finally, if all this is not enough, consider the fact that smoking will absolutely reduce the quality and quantity of your sex life. The quality ebbs as endurance and general health decreases. The quantity will decline with the premature blockage of the abdominal aorta and internal hypogastric arteries which deliver blood to the sex organs.

All in all, there is no rationalization for smoking. Once again, if you smoke—quit!

Exposure to the Sun

While suntans are certainly attractive and fashionable, acquiring them is directly related to the development of skin cancer. (Light-skinned, blue-eyed people are more likely to be affected than those with darker complexions.) Although, in some cases, tanning is a direct result of a person's occupation, such as farming, a large percentage of people purposely spend time in the sun to look more healthy. Unfortunately, in reality, it might not only have the opposite effect, the results can be fatal.

Most of the related malignancies are associated with either the basal or squamous skin cells. Both have a very high cure rate as they are visible and more easily diagnosed in the early stages and tend to remain localized. These often take the form of a pale wax-like, pearly nodule or a red, scaly, sharply-outlined patch. Malignant melanoma, however, is deadly and has a tendency to spread and grow rapidly in its early course. It often starts as a small mole-like growth that increases in size, changes color, becomes ulcerated and bleeds easily from slight injury.

Like malignancies caused by smoking, skin cancers are preventable. The first step is to make a point of not purposely attaining a tan. Second, use protective clothing, a wide-brimmed hat and a good sunscreen preparation when you must be outdoors in the sunshine.

Alcohol

Alcohol consumption can also be modified to prevent cancer. Heavy drinkers show higher incidence of oral cancers and cancers of the larynx, throat, esophagus, and liver. It is estimated that a reduced alcohol intake by the general population might bring a 30% reduction in 20 years.

Industrial Hazards

Exposure to a number of industrial agents (nickel, chromate, asbestos, vinyl chloride, etc.) will place a person at increased risk. Since one of the major target organs of industrial chemicals is the lungs, it is vital that people who work around these agents do not smoke. For example, a smoker exposed to asbestos fibers has a lung cancer risk 60 times higher than an individual who does not smoke and is not around asbestos.

Nutrition

There is extensive research underway to evaluate the exact relationship of nutrition to cancer. While there is no doubt that one exists, a direct cause and effect has not yet been proven. There are a number of facts based on statistical evidence, however, and these should definitely be considered.

To begin with, risk may be decreased by simply dieting off excess weight. Obese individuals show increased incidence of breast, uterine and colon cancer. It is also known that our western diet lacks fiber and that this absence is implicated in colon cancer. Keep in mind that high fiber foods such as vegetables, fresh fruits and cereals are also low in fat and high in vitamins.

The National Cancer Institute and The American Cancer Society feel that diets rich in Vitamin A, Vitamin C, and a precursor of Vitamin A called beta-carotene, might reduce the risk of certain cancers. Foods containing these elements include dark green, leafy vegetables, other green vegetables as well as those that are red, yellow and orange, and of course, citrus fruits. Members of the cabbage family, called cruciferous vegetables, are also important. These include broccoli, brussel sprouts, cauliflower, etc.

So, in summary, it's important to make a conscious effort, both when shopping, and when dining out, to choose primarily healthy foods. Start your day with fruit—an apple or orange—instead of a donut or turnover. Look for low-fat dairy products rather than those consisting of whole milk. Instead of white bread, which is composed of refined flours, eat those made with 100% whole grain flours such as whole wheat. Use vegetable oil when you fry foods and pick lean cuts of meat. Use methods such as baking, steaming, roasting or your microwave when you cook. These add no fat.

The Immune System

Many doctors and researchers feel that cancers develop during a daily turnover of several billion cells as new ones replace those that are dying off. While some of the replacements will naturally be abnormal, for the most part they are mutants which create no problems. However, a few do have cancer-causing potential and seem to develop at rather frequent intervals. The reason that we do not all die of cancer is that our bodies contain a remarkable immune system that first recognizes abnormal cells, then attacks and destroys them. (This is also true for all other foreign invaders, such as viruses or bacteria). The immune system is highly complex and is being better understood as time goes on. One important aspect is that there are specific steps that we can each take to strengthen it and make it work more efficiently.

Iron deficiency will depress the immune system. This is not an uncommon problem, particularly in premenopausal women. Therefore, it's important to eat foods rich in iron such as lean meats, leafy green vegetables, shellfish and fruits and vegetables rich in Vitamin C.

Strong sunlight also adversely affects the immune

system so again, use a sunscreen when exposure is unavoidable.

We all know that regular exercise has outstanding benefits to the muscles and the respiratory and circulatory systems. The psychiatric profession also advocates it for its beneficial effects in the areas of mental illness and its positive influence on a person's attitude. In addition to all this, exercise improves our immune system. Almost any program of regular physical activity is good for you, provided it is matched with your age and physical condition. You should probably consult your physician about a good exercise regimen suited to your particular needs.

Stress

Stress, particularly in today's society, is unavoidable, and unfortunately, it affects the immune system along with other aspects of our well being. I could write another book on the effects of stress, but will simply caution you to try to be conscious of what causes it in your own life. By trying to handle situations so as to minimize it you will strengthen your immune system as well.

13
Chemotherapeutic Agents

I strongly believe, and psychological studies confirm, that the more a woman knows about her disease, its diagnosis and its treatment, the more beneficial it is to her. We all fear the unknown, so as a patient develops an understanding of what she is facing, her anxiety level begins to recede. I have often been told by my patients that they can deal with the treatment, but they just want to understand what is happening.

With this in mind, I have included several of the more commonly used chemotherapeutic agents used in treating cancer of the breast. Chemotherapy is not to be taken lightly, and must be administered only under the care and supervision of a medical oncologist. While this physician will explain the possible side effects, I feel that also reading about it will enable you to develop a deeper understanding of the processes involved. There may be some points that were not clear when they were explained, but will make more sense when you read about them. Knowledge of the complications may also give rise to further questions for the physician.

Each of the following entries contains the generic name of the drug and also proprietary names and pronunciation. More common side effects are listed as well.

You will notice that the first page consists of a combination of drugs preceded by an acronym. These acronyms are for convenience since usually anywhere from three to five drugs are used simultaneously during chemotherapy. For example, CMF is a combination of cyclophosphamide, methotrexate and fluorouracil.

At the time of this writing, no single combination has been proven superior. This may change in the near future as there are a number of clinical studies currently underway that will evaluate several newer drugs currently in the investigative stage.

ANTICANCER DRUG COMBINATIONS

ABVD:	A combination of doxorubicin + bleomycin + vinblastine + dacarbazine.
CHOP:	A combination of cyclophosphamide + doxorubicin + vincristine + prednisone.
CMF:	A combination of cyclophosphamide + methotrexate + fluorouracil.
COPP:	A combination of cyclophosphamide + vincristine + procarbazine + prednisone.
CVP:	A combination of cyclophosphamide + vincristine + prednisone.
CY-VA-DIC:	A combination of cyclophosphamide + vincristine + doxorubicin + dacarbazine.
FAC:	A combination of fluorouracil + doxorubicin + cyclophosphamide.
FAM:	A combination of fluorouracil + doxorubicin + mitomycin.
MOPP:	A combination of mechlorethamine + vincristine + procarbazine + prednisone.
MPL + PRED:	A combination of melphalan + prednisone.
MTX + MP + CTX:	A combination of methotrexate + mercaptopurine + cyclophosphamide.
PVB:	See VBP
VAC:	A combination of vincristine + dactinomycin + cyclophosphamide.
VBP:	A combination of vinblastine + bleomycin + cisplatin.
VP-L-Asparaginase:	A combination of vincristine + prednisone + asparaginase.

Refer to the individual drug listing for information on each medicine in these drug combinations.

CHEMOTHERAPEUTIC AGENTS

ASPARAGINASE

Pronunciation: A-SPARE-a-gin-ase

Brand Name: Elspar (TM)

How Given: Injection

Special Precautions:
Your physician may order additional fluid intake to prevent kidney and bladder problems.

Side Effects Which . . .

- **Require Immediate Medical Attention:**
  Difficulty in breathing; joint pain; puffy face; skin rash or itching; stomach pain with severe nausea and vomiting.

- **Require Medical Attention As Soon As Possible:**
  Yellowing of eyes and skin; confusion; drowsiness; fever, chills, or sore throat; flank or stomach pain; hallucinations; depression; nervousness; sores in mouth or on lips; swelling of feet or lower legs; tiredness; unusually frequent urination; unusual thirst; convulsions; severe headaches.

- **Require Medical Attention If They Occur After Treatment Is Completed:**
  Stomach pain with nausea and vomiting.

- **Require No Medical Attention (Unless Severe Or Prolonged):**
  Headache; loss of appetite; nausea and vomiting; stomach cramps; weight loss.

BLEOMYCIN

Pronunciation: Blee-oh-My-sin

Brand Name: Blenoxane (TM)

How Given: IV or IM Injection

Side Effects Which . . .

- **Require Immediate Medical Attention:**
  Fever and chills occurring within three to six hours after dosing; faintness; confusion; sweating; wheezing.

- **Require Medical Attention As Soon As Possible:**
  Cough; Shortness of breath; sores in mouth and on lips.

- **Require Medical Attention If They Occur After Treatment Is Completed:**
  Cough, shortness of breath.
- **Require No Medical Attention (Unless Severe Or Prolonged):**
  Darkening or thickening of skin; itching of skin; skin rash or colored bumps on fingertips, elbows, or palms; skin redness or tenderness; swelling of the fingers; vomiting and loss of appetite.

Note: Side effects on the lungs (i.e., cough and shortness of breath) are more likely if you smoke. These are most common in older patients.

BULSUFAN

Pronunciation: Byoo-SUL-fan
Brand Name: Myleran (TM)
How Given: Orally
Special Precautions:
Your physician may order additional fluid intake to prevent kidney and bladder problems.

Side Effects Which . . .
- **Require Medical Attention As Soon As Possible:**
  Fever, chills, or sore throat; unusual bleeding or bruising; cough, side or stomach pain; joint pain; shortness of breath; swelling of feet or lower legs.
- **Require Medical Attention If They Occur After Treatment Is Completed:**
  Fever, cough or shortness of breath; unusual bleeding or bruising.
- **Require No Medical Attention (Unless Severe Or Prolonged):**
  Darkening of the skin; confusion; diarrhea; dizziness; loss of appetite; nausea and vomiting; unusual tiredness.

CARMUSTINE

Pronunciation: Kar-MUS-teen
Brand Name: BiCNU (TM)
Commonly referred to as BCNU
How Given: IV Injection

Special Precautions:
If drug accidentally seeps out of the vein, it may damage tissues and cause scarring. Immediately inform the doctor or nurse of redness, pain or swelling at the IV site.

Side Effects Which . . .

- **Require Medical Attention As Soon As Possible:**
  Cough; fever; chills or sore throat; shortness of breath; unusual bleeding or bruising; flushing of face; sores in mouth and on lips; unusual tiredness or weakness; swelling of feet or lower legs; unusual decrease in urination.

- **Require Medical Attention If They Occur After Treatment Is Completed:**
  Cough; fever, chills or sore throat; shortness of breath; unusual bleeding or bruising;

- **Require No Medical Attention (Unless Severe Or Prolonged):**
  Nausea and vomiting lasting no more than six hours; discoloration of skin along the vein of injection; diarrhea; difficulty in swallowing; difficulty in walking; dizziness; loss of appetite; loss of hair; skin rash and itching.

  Note: Side effects on the lungs (i.e. cough and shortness of breath) are more likely if you smoke.

CHLORAMBUCIL

Pronunciation: Klor-AM-byoo-sill

Brand Name: Leukeran (TM)

How Given: Orally

Special Precautions:
Your physician may order additional fluid intake to prevent kidney and bladder problems.

Side Effects Which . . .

- **Require Medical Attention As Soon As Possible:**
  Fever, chills, or sore throat; sores in mouth and on lips; unusual bleeding or bruising; side or stomach pain; joint pain; skin rash; swelling of feet or lower legs; convulsions; cough; shortness of breath; yellowing of eyes and skin.

- **Require Medical Attention If They Occur After Treatment Is Completed:**

Cough; fever, chills, or sore throat; shortness of breath, unusual bleeding or bruising.

CISPLATIN

Pronunciation: SIS-pla-tin

Brand Name: Platinol (TM)

Commonly referred to as Cis-platinum

How Given: IV Injection

Special Precautions:
Your physician may order additional fluid intake to prevent kidney or bladder problems.

If drug accidentally seeps out of the vein, it may damage tissues and cause scarring. Immediately inform the doctor or nurse of redness, pain or swelling at the IV site.

Side Effects Which . . .

- **Require Immediate Medical Attention:**
  Swelling of face; unusually fast heartbeat; wheezing.
- **Require Medical Attention As Soon As Possible:**
  Difficulty in hearing; fever, chills, or sore throat; side or stomach pain; joint pain; ringing in ears; swelling of feet or lower legs; unusual bleeding or bruising; loss of taste; unusual tiredness or weakness; numbness or tingling in the fingers, toes or face; blurred vision.
- **Require Medical Attention If They Occur After Treatment Is Completed:**
  Difficulty in hearing; fever, chills or sore throat; ringing in ears; swelling of feet or lower legs; unusual bleeding or bruising; unusual decrease in urination.
- **Require No Medical Attention (Unless Severe Or Prolonged):**
  Nausea and vomiting.

    Note: Hearing problems are more likely to occur in children.

CLOPHOSPHAMIDE

Pronunciation: Sye-kloe-FOSS-fa-mide

Brand Name: Cytoxan (TM)

How Given: Orally or by Injections

Special Precautions:
Your physician may order additional fluid intake to prevent kidney or bladder problems.

If you are receiving this medicine by injection, check with your doctor if you notice redness, swelling, or pain at the IV site.

Check with your doctor immediately if you notice blood in your urine after you have stopped taking this medication.

Side Effects Which . . .

- **Require Immediate Medical Attention:**
  Blood in urine; painful urination.

- **Require Medical Attention As Soon As Possible:**
  Dizziness, confusion, or agitation; fever, chills or sore throat; missed menstrual periods; tiredness; cough; side or stomach pain; joint pain; shortness of breath; swelling of feet or lower legs; unusual bleeding or bruising; unusually fast heartbeat; black, tarry stools; sores in mouth and on lips; unusually frequent urination; unusual thirst; yellow eyes and skin.

- **Require No Medical Attention (Unless Severe Or Prolonged):**
  Darkening of skin and fingernails; loss of appetite; loss of hair; nausea and vomiting.

CYTARABINE

Pronunciation: Sye-TARE-a-been

Brand Name: Cytosar-U (TM)

Commonly referred to as Ara-C

How Given: Injections

Special Precautions:
Your physician may order additional fluid intake to prevent kidney or bladder problems.

Side Effects Which . . .

- **Require Medical Attention As Soon As Possible:**
  Fever, chills, and sore throat; unusual bleeding or bruising; side or stomach pain; joint pain; numbness or tingling in fingers, toes, or face; sores in mouth and on lips; swelling of feet and lower legs; tiredness; black, tarry stools; difficulty in swallowing; fainting spells; general feeling of body discomfort or weakness; heartburn; irregular heartbeat; pain at place of injection; reddened eyes; shortness of breath; skin rash; unusual decrease in urination; yellowing of eyes and skin.

- **Require Medical Attention If They Occur After Treatment Is Completed:**
  Fever and chills; sore throat; unusual bleeding or bruising.
- **Require No Medical Attention (Unless Severe Or Prolonged):**
  Loss of appetite; nausea and vomiting.

DECARBAZINE

Pronunciation: Da-KAR-ba-zeen

Brand Name: DTIC-Dome (TM)

How Given: IV Injection

Special Precautions:
If drug accidentally seeps out of the vein, it may damage tissues and cause scarring. Immediately inform the doctor or nurse of redness, pain or swelling at the IV site.

Side Effects Which . . .
- **Require Medical Attention As Soon As Possible:**
  Fever, chills, or sore throat; unusual bleeding or bruising; sores in mouth and on lips.
- **Require Medical Attention If They Occur After Treatment Is Completed:**
  Fever, chills, or sore throat; unusual bleeding or bruising.
- **Require No Medical Attention (Unless Severe Or Prolonged):**
  Loss of appetite; nausea and vomiting.

DACTINOMYCIN

Pronunciation: Dak-ti-neo-MYE-sin

Brand Name: Cosmegen (TM)

How Given: IV Injection

Special Precautions:
If drug accidentally seeps out of the vein, it may damage tissues and cause scarring. Immediately inform the doctor or nurse of redness, pain or swelling at the IV site.

Side Effects Which . . .
- **Require Immediate Medical Attention:**
  Fever, chills, sore throat; unusual bleeding or bruising.

- **Require Medical Attention As Soon As Possible:**
  Black, tarry stools; continuing diarrhea; continuing stomach pain; difficulty in swallowing; heartburn; sores in mouth and on lips; joint pain; swelling of feet or lower legs; yellowing of eyes and skin.
- **Require Medical Attention If They Occur After Treatment Is Completed:**
  Black, tarry stools; diarrhea; fever, chills or sore throat; sores in mouth and on lips; stomach pain; unusual bleeding or bruising; yellowing of eyes and skin.
- **Require No Medical Attention (Unless Severe Or Prolonged):**
  Darkening of skin; loss of hair (may include eyebrows); nausea and vomiting; reddening of skin; skin rash or acne; tiredness.

DAUNORUBICIN

Pronunciation: Daw-noe-roo-bi-sin

Brand Name: Cerubidine (TM)

How Given: IV Injection

Special Precautions:

If drug accidentally seeps out of the vein, it may damage tissues and cause scarring. Immediately inform the doctor or nurse of redness, pain or swelling at the IV site.

Your physician may order additional fluid intake to prevent kidney and bladder problems.

Side Effects Which . . .

- **Require Immediate Medical Attention:**
  Irregular heartbeat; pain at the places of injection; shortness of breath; swelling of feet and lower legs.
- **Require Medical Attention As Soon As Possible:**
  Fever, chills or sore throat; sores in mouth and on lips; stomach pain; unusual bleeding or bruising; skin rash or itching.
- **Require Medical Attention If They Occur After Treatment Is Completed:**
  Swelling of feet and lower legs; irregular heartbeat; shortness of breath.
- **Require No Medical Attention (Unless Severe Or Prolonged):**
  Loss of hair; nausea and vomiting (mild); darkening or redness of skin; diarrhea.

Note: Causes urine to turn reddish which may stain clothes. This is not blood. It is normal and lasts for only one or two days after each dose is given.

DOXORUBICIN

Pronunciation: Dox-oh-ROO-bi-sin

Brand Name: Adriamycin (TM)

How Given: IV Injection

Special Precautions:
Your physician may order additional fluid intake to prevent kidney and bladder problems.

If drug accidentally seeps out of the vein, it may damage tissues and cause scarring. Immediately inform the doctor or nurse of redness, pain or swelling at the IV site.

Side Effects Which . . .

- **Require Immediate Medical Attention:**
  Unusually fast or irregular heartbeat; pain at place of injection; shortness of breath; swelling of feet and lower legs; wheezing.
- **Require Medical Attention As Soon As Possible:**
  Fever, chills, or sore throat; sores in mouth and on lips; side or stomach pain; joint pain; unusual bleeding or bruising; skin rash or itching.
- **Require Medical Attention If They Occur After Treatment Is Completed:**
  Irregular heartbeat; shortness of breath; swelling of feet and lower legs.
- **Require No Medical Attention (Unless Severe Or Prolonged):**
  Loss of hair; nausea or vomiting; reddish urine; darkening of soles, palms or nails.

Note: Causes urine to turn reddish which may stain clothes. This is not blood. It is normal and lasts for only one or two days after each dose is given.

FLOXURODINE

Pronunciation: Flox-YOOR-i-deen

Brand Name: FUDR (TM)

How Given: Injection

Special Precautions:
If nausea, vomiting, and/or stomach pain occurs, inform your physician immediately.

Side Effects Which . . .
- **Require Immediate Medical Attention:**
  Diarrhea; sores in mouth and on lips; stomach pain or cramps; black tarry stools; heartburn; fever, chills, or sore throat; nausea and vomiting; swelling or soreness of tongue; difficulty walking; unusual bleeding or bruising; yellowing of eyes and skin.

FLOUROURACIL

Pronunciation: Floor-oh-YOOR-a-sill
Brand Name: Adrucil (TM)
How Given: Injection

Side Effects Which . . .
- **Require Immediate Medical Attention:**
  Diarrhea; fever, chills, or sore throat; heartburn; sores in mouth and on lips; black, tarry stools; nausea and severe vomiting; stomach cramps; unusual bleeding or bruising.
- **Require Medical Attention As Soon As Possible:**
  Chest pain; cough; difficulty with balance; shortness of breath.
- **Require Medical Attention If They Occur After Treatment Is Completed:**
  Fever, chills, sore throat; unusual bleeding or bruising.
- **Require No Medical Attention (Unless Severe Or Prolonged):**
  Loss of appetite; loss of hair; nausea and vomiting; skin rash and itching, weakness.

HYDROXYUREA

Pronunciation: Hye-DROX-ee-yoo-REE-ah
Brand Name: Hydrea (TM)
How Given: Orally
Special Precautions:
Your physician may order additional fluid intake to prevent kidney and bladder problems.

Side Effects Which . . .
- **Require Immediate Medical Attention:**
  Fever, chills, or sore throat; sores in mouth and on lips;

unusual bleeding or bruising; convulsions; dizziness; side or stomach pain; hallucinations; headache; joint pain; confusion; swelling of feet or lower legs.

Note: The above are more likely to occur in children and in elderly patients.

- **Require Medical Attention If They Occur After Treatment is Completed:**
  Unusual bleeding or bruising; fever, chills, or sore throat;

- **Require No Medical Attention (Unless Severe Or Prolonged):**
  Diarrhea; drowsiness; loss of appetite; nausea; vomiting.

- **Require Medical Attention If They Occur After Treatment Is Completed:**
  Fever, chills, or sore throat; unusual bleeding or bruising.

- **Require No Medical Attention (Unless Severe Or Prolonged):**
  Nausea and vomiting.

LOMOSTINE

Pronunciation: Loe-MUS-teen

Brand Name: CeeNU (TM)

Commonly referred to as CCNU

How Given: Orally

Special Precautions:
Possibility of two or more different types of capsules in the container. It is important to take all the medication as one dose in order to receive the right amount of medicine.

Side Effects Which . . .

- **Require Immediate Medical Attention:**
  Fever, chills, sore throat; unusual bleeding or bruising; awkwardness, confusion, slurred speech; sores in mouth and/or on lips; swelling of feet or lower legs; unusual decrease in urination; unusual tiredness or weakness; yellowing of eyes and skin; cough or shortness of breath.

- **Require Medical Attention If They Occur After Treatment Is Completed:**
  Fever, chills, sore throat; unusual bleeding or bruising.

- **Require No Medical Attention (Unless Severe Or Prolonged):**
  Loss of appetite; nausea and vomiting (usually lasts less than 24 hours); darkening of the skin; diarrhea; loss of hair; skin rash and itching.

MECHLORETHAMINE

Pronunciation: Me-klor-ETH-a-meen

Brand Name: Mustargen (TM)

Commonly referred to as Nitrogen Mustard

How Given: IV Injection

Special Precautions:
Your physician may order additional fluid intake to prevent kidney and bladder problems.

If drug accidentally seeps out of the vein, it may damage tissues and cause scarring. Immediately inform the doctor or nurse of redness, pain or swelling at the IV site.

Side Effects Which . . .

- **Require Immediate Medical Attention:**
  Wheezing.
- **Require Medical Attention As Soon As Possible:**
  Fever, chills, or sore throat; missed menstrual periods; painful rash; unusual bleeding or bruising; dizziness; side and stomach pain; joint pain; loss of hearing; ringing in ears; swelling of feet or lower legs; black, tarry stools; itching; numbness; tingling or burning of fingers, toes, face; shortness of breath; yellowing of eyes and skin.

MELPHALAN

Pronunciation: MEL-fa-lan

Brand Name: Alkeran (TM)

How Given: Orally

Special Precautions:
Your physician may order additional fluid intake to prevent kidney and bladder problems.

Side Effects Which . . .

- **Require Immediate Medical Attention:**
  Sudden skin rash and itching.

- **Require Medical Attention As Soon As Possible:**
  Black, tarry stools; fever, chills, or sore throat; unusual bleeding or bruising; side or stomach pain; joint pain, sores in mouth and on lips; swelling of feet or lower legs.
- **Require Medical Attention If They Occur After Treatment Is Completed:**
  Fever, chills, or sore throat; unusual bleeding or bruising.
- **Require No Medical Attention (Unless Severe Or Prolonged):**
  Nausea or vomiting.

MERCAPTOPURINE

Pronunciation: Mer-kap-toe-PYOOR-een

Brand Name: Purinethol (TM)

How Given: Orally

Special Precautions:
Your physician may order additional fluid intake to prevent kidney and bladder problems.

Avoid alcoholic beverages unless approved by your doctor. Alcohol may increase the harmful effects of this medicine.

Side Effects Which . . .
- **Require Medical Attention As Soon As Possible:**
  Fever, chills, sore throat; unusual bleeding or bruising; unusual tiredness or weakness; yellowing of eyes and skin; loss of appetite; side or stomach pain; joint pain; nausea and vomiting; swelling of feet or lower legs; black tarry stools; sores in mouth and on lips.
- **Require Medical Attention If They Occur After Treatment Is Completed:**
  Chills or sore throat; unusual bleeding or bruising; yellowing of eyes and skin;

METHOTREXATE

Pronunciation: Meth-o-TREX-ate

Brand Name: Mexate (TM)

How Given: Orally or Injection

Special Precautions:
Your physician may order additional fluid intake to prevent kidney and bladder problems.

Avoid alcoholic beverages unless approved by your doctor. Alcohol may increase the harmful effects of this medicine.

Do not take aspirin or any other preparations containing aspirin or salicylate compounds without first checking with your doctor as they may increase the drug's effects.

Side Effects Which . . .
- **Require Immediate Medical Attention:**
  Black, tarry stools; bloody vomit; diarrhea; sores in mouth and on lips; stomach pain.
- **Require Medical Attention As Soon As Possible:**
  Fever, chills, or sore throat; unusual bleeding or bruising; blood in urine; blurred vision; confusion; convulsions or seizures; cough; dark urine; dizziness; drowsiness; headache; joint pain; shortness of breath; swelling of feet or lower legs; unusual tiredness or weakness; yellowing of eyes and skin.
- **Require Medical Attention If They Occur After Treatment Is Completed:**
  Blurred vision; convulsions or seizures; dizziness; drowsiness; headache; confusion; unusual tiredness or weakness.
- **Require No Medical Attention (Unless Severe Or Prolonged):**
  Loss of appetite; nausea or vomiting.

Note: The above side effects may be more likely to occur in very young or very old patients.

MITOMYCIN

Pronunciation: Mye-toe-MYE-sin

Brand Name: Mutamycin (TM)

How Given: IV Injection

Special Precautions:
If drug accidentally seeps out of the vein, it may damage tissues and cause scarring. Immediately inform the doctor or nurse of redness, pain or swelling at the IV site.

Side Effects Which . . .
- **Require Immediate Medical Attention:**
  Blood in urine.
- **Require Medical Attention As Soon As Possible:**
  Fever, chills, sore throat; unusual bleeding or bruising;

cough; decreased urination; shortness of breath; sores in mouth and on lips; swelling of feet or lower legs; bloody vomit.
- **Require Medical Attention If They Occur After Treatment Is Completed:**
Fever, chills, or sore throat; unusual bleeding or bruising; decreased urination; shortness of breath; swelling of feet or lower legs.
- **Require No Medical Attention (Unless Severe Or Prolonged):**
Loss of appetite; nausea and vomiting.

MITOTANE

Pronunciation: MYE-toe-tane

Brand Name: Lysodren (TM)

How Given: Orally

Special Precautions:
May cause some people to become dizzy, drowsy, or less alert than normal. Use extreme caution before driving, using machines, or performing other jobs that require alertness.

Will add to the effect of alcohol and other central nervous system (CNS) depressants (medicines that slow down the nervous system, possibly causing drowsiness). Check with your doctor before using alcohol or other CNS depressants while you are taking this medicine.

Contact your doctor immediately if you are injured, infected or contract illness of any kind.

Side Effects Which . . .
- **Require Immediate Medical Attention:**
Stop taking this medicine and check with your doctor if the following side effects occur: Darkening of skin; diarrhea; dizziness; drowsiness; loss of appetite; depression; nausea and vomiting; skin rash; tiredness.
- **Require Medical Attention As Soon As Possible:**
Blood in urine; blurred or double vision; shortness of breath; wheezing.

PLICAMYCIN

Pronunciation: Plye-ka-MYE-sin

Brand Name: Mithracin and Mithramycin (TM)

How Given: Injection

Special Precautions:
Do not take aspirin or any other preparations containing aspirin or salicylate compounds without first checking with your doctor as they may increase the drug's effects.

Side Effects Which . . .

- **Require Immediate Medical Attention:**
  Bloody or black, tarry stools; flushing, redness or swelling of face; skin rash or small red spots on skin; sore throat and fever; unexplained nosebleed; unusual bleeding or bruising; vomiting of blood.

- **Require Medical Attention As Soon As Possible:**
  Nausea or vomiting; drowsiness; fever; headache; redness; depression; pain; soreness or swelling at place of injection; unusual tiredness or weakness.

- **Require Medical Attention If They Occur After Treatment Is Completed:**
  Bloody or black, tarry stools; small red spots on skin; sore throat and fever; unexplained nosebleed; unusual bleeding or bruising; vomiting of blood.

- **Require No Medical Attention (Unless Severe Or Prolonged):**
  Diarrhea; irritation or soreness of mouth; appetite loss.

PREDNISONE

Pronunciation: PRED-ni-sone

Brand Name: Deltasone (TM), Metocirten (TM), Orasone (TM)

How Given: Orally

Special Precautions:
Your doctor may want you to follow a low-salt and/or a potassium-rich diet if you will be using the drug for an extended period of time.

Before undergoing any kind of surgery (including dental) or emergency treatment, inform the doctor in charge that you are taking this drug.

Diabetic patients should note that this medicine may affect blood sugar levels. You should check with your doctor if you detect a change in your urine sugar tests or have any other questions.

Side Effects Which . . .

- **Require Medical Attention As Soon As Possible:**
  Decreased or blurred vision; frequent urination; in-

creased thirst; rash, acne, or other skin problems; back or rib pain; bloody or black, tarry stools; filling- or rounding out of the face; irregular heartbeats; menstrual problems; depression; mood or mental changes; muscle cramps or pains; muscle weakness; nausea or vomiting; seeing halos around lights; sore throat and fever; continued stomach pain or burning; swelling of feet or lower legs; unusual tiredness or weakness; wounds that do not heal.

- **Require Medical Attention If They Occur After Treatment Is Completed:**
Pain in abdomen, stomach, or back; dizziness or fainting; fever; continued loss of appetite; muscle or joint pain; nausea or vomiting; shortness of breath; frequent or continuing headaches; unusual tiredness or weakness; unusual weight loss.

- **Require No Medical Attention (Unless Severe Or Prolonged):**
Indigestion; false sense of well-being; increase in appetite; nervousness or restlessness; trouble in sleeping; weight gain.

Note: Your body may take time to adjust following cessation of treatment.

PROCARBAZINE

Pronunciation: Pro-KAR-ba-zeen

Brand Name: Matulane (TM) and Natulan (TM)

How Given: Orally

Special Precautions:

Immediately check with your doctor or hospital emergency room if severe headache, stiff neck, chest pains, or rapid heartbeat, with nausea and vomiting, occur while you are taking this medicine. These may be symptoms of a serious high blood pressure reaction and should have a doctor's attention.

Procarbazine can cause very dangerous reactions when combined with certain foods, drinks or other medicines. Do not . . .

- eat foods with high tyramine content (most common in foods that are aged to increase their flavor), such as cheeses, sour cream, yogurt, pickled herring, chicken livers, soy sauce, canned figs, raisins, bananas, avocados, broad bean pods (fava beans), yeast extracts, or meats prepared with tenderizers.

- drink alcoholic beverages, including beer and wines (particularly Chianti and hearty red wines).
- take any other medicine unless prescribed by your doctor. This especially applies to over-the-counter medicines such as those for colds (including nose drops), cough, asthma, hay fever, alertness or appetite control.

For at least two weeks after completion of treatment, you must continue to observe cautionary rules concerning food, drink and other medication as the drug may continue to react with certain foods or other medicines for up to 14 days.

This medicine may cause some people to become drowsy or less alert than normal. Determine your own reaction before you drive, run machinery or perform other tasks that require alertness.

Immediately stop taking this medicine and check with your physician if the following side effects occur: chest pains; rapid or irregular heartbeat; severe headache; stiff neck.

Side Effects Which . . .

- **Require Medical Attention As Soon As Possible:**
  Black, tarry stools; bloody vomit; convulsions; cough; fever, chills, or sore throat; hallucinations, missed menstrual periods; shortness of breath; thickening of bronchial secretions; continuing tiredness or weakness; unusual bleeding or bruising; diarrhea; sores in mouth and on lips; tingling or numbness of the fingers or toes; unsteadiness or awkwardness; yellowing of the eyes or skin; fainting; skin rash; hives; itching; wheezing.
- **Require No Medical Attention (Unless Severe Or Prolonged):**
  Drowsiness, muscle or joint pain; muscle twitching; nervousness; nightmares; nausea and vomiting; sweating; sleeplessness; tiredness; weakness; darkening of the skin; dizziness or lightheadedness when getting up from a lying or sitting position; Warmth and/or redness in face.

STREPTOZOCIN

Pronunciation: Strep-toe-ZOE-sin
Brand Name: Zanosar (TM)
How Given: IV Injection

Special Precautions:

Your physician may order additional fluid intake to prevent kidney and bladder problems.

If drug accidentally seeps out of the vein, it may damage tissues and cause scarring. Immediately inform the doctor or nurse of redness, pain or swelling at the IV site.

Side Effects Which . . .

- **Require Immediate Medical Attention:**
  Anxiety, nervousness, or shakiness; chills, cold sweats, or cool, pale skin; drowsiness or unusual tiredness or weakness; headache; pain or redness at place of injection; unusual hunger, unusually fast pulse.

- **Require Medical Attention As Soon As Possible:**
  Swelling of feet or lower legs; unusual decrease in urination; fever, chills, or sore throat; unusual bleeding or bruising; yellowing of eyes or skin.

- **Require Medical Attention If They Occur After Treatment Is Completed:**
  Swelling of feet or lower legs; unusual decrease in urination.

- **Require No Medical Attention (Unless Severe Or Prolonged):**
  Nausea and vomiting (unusual occurring within two hours following dosage); diarrhea

VINBLASTINE

Pronunciation: Vin-BLAS-teen

Brand Name: Velban (TM)

How Given: IV Injection

Special Precautions:

Your physician may order additional fluid intake to prevent kidney and bladder problems.

If drug accidentally seeps out of the vein, it may damage tissues and cause scarring. Immediately inform the doctor or nurse of redness, pain or swelling at the IV site.

Side Effects Which . . .

- **Require Medical Attention As Soon As Possible:**
  Fever, chills, or sore throat; side or stomach pain; joint pain; swelling of feet and lower legs; unusual bleeding or bruising; black, tarry stool; difficulty in walking; jaw

pain; dizziness; double vision; drooping eyelids; sores in mouth and on lips; headache; depression; numbness or ringing in fingers and toes; pain in fingers and toes; pain in testicles; weakness.

- **Require No Medical Attention (Unless Severe Or Prolonged):**
  Loss of hair; muscle pain; nausea and vomiting.

VINCRISTINE

Pronunciation: Vin-KRIS-teen

Brand Name: Oncovin (TM)

How Given: IV Injection

Special Precautions:

Your physician may order additional fluid intake to prevent kidney and bladder problems.

Vincristine frequently causes constipation and stomach cramps. Your doctor may want you to take a laxative or stool softener; however, do not take these medicines on your own without prior approval.

Side Effects Which . . .

- **Require Medical Attention As Soon As Possible:**
  Blurred or double vision; constipation; side or stomach pain; difficulty walking; drooping eyelids; headache; jaw pain; joint pain; numbness or tingling in fingers and toes; pain in fingers and toes; pain in testicles; stomach cramps; swelling of feet or lower legs; weakness; painful or difficult urination; agitation; bed-wetting; confusion; convulsions; dizziness or lightheadedness when getting up from a sitting or lying position; hallucinations; lack of sweating; loss of appetite; depression; seizures; trouble sleeping; unconsciousness; unusual decrease or increase in urination; cough; fever; chills; sore throat; shortness of breath; sores in mouth and on lips; unusual bleeding or bruising.

- **Require No Medical Attention (Unless Severe Or Prolonged):**
  Loss of hair; bloating; diarrhea; weight loss; nausea and vomiting; skin rash.

- **Note:**   Nervous system effects may be more likely to occur in older patients.

Glossary

Adjuvant Chemotherapy	The use of drugs in addition to surgery and/or radiation to treat cancer.
Alopecia	The loss of hair from the body and/or the scalp.
Anemia	Low red blood cell count; symptoms include shortness of breath, lack of energy, and fatigue.
Anesthesia	Entire or partial loss of feeling or sensation resulting from the administration of drugs or gases.
Anorexia	Absence or loss of appetite for food.
Antiemetic	A medicine that prevents or controls vomiting.
Benign	Not cancerous
Benign Tumor	A noncancerous growth that does not spread to other parts of the body. Recovery is favorable with treatment.
Blood Count	The number of red blood cells, white cells, and platelets in a given sample of blood.
Bone Marrow	The inner spongy tissue of a bone where red blood cells, white cells, and platelets are formed.
Breast Enlargement	An operation in which an implant is inserted under normal breast tissues.
Breast Implant	A round or teardrop-shaped sac inserted in the body to restore a breast form.
Breast Prosthesis	An artificial breast form that can be worn under clothing after a mastectomy.
Breast Reduction	An operation in which breast skin and tissue are removed and the nipple is moved up onto the newly contoured breast.

BSE—Breast Self-Examination	Monthly examination of the breast by the woman herself.
Cancer	A general term for more than 100 diseases characterized by abnormal and uncontrolled growth of cells. The resulting mass, or tumor, can invade and destroy surrounding normal tissues. Cancer cells from the tumor can spread through the blood or lymph (the clear fluid that bathes body cells) to start new cancers in other parts of the body.
Catheter	A tube used for injection or withdrawal of fluid.
Cell	The basic structure of living tissues; all plants and animals are made up of one or more cells.
Chemotherapy	Treatment with drugs to destroy cancer cells. Most often used to supplement surgery and/or radiation therapy.
Combination Chemotherapy	The use of several drugs at the same time or in a particular order to treat cancer.
Cyst	A fluid-filled mass that is usually harmless and can be removed by aspiration.
Discharge	Clear, milky, or bloody fluid coming from the nipple.
Duct	A structure in the breast through which milk passes from glands to the nipple.
Estrogen	A female hormone produced by the woman's ovaries and adrenal glands.
Fat	Tissue that helps give shape to the breast, similar to fat in other parts of the body.
Fibrocystic Disease	A general term for a number of non-cancerous breast conditions usually involving lumpiness and/or pain.
Gastrointestinal (GI)	Having to do with the digestive tract, which includes the stomach and the intestines.
Immunotherapy	Treatment by stimulation of the body's immune defense system. Doctors are doing research on immunotherapy as a possible treatment for cancer.
Infusion	The process of putting fluids into the vein by letting them drip slowly through a tube.
Injection	The use of a syringe to "push" fluids into the body; often called a "shot".

Intramuscular (IM)	Into a muscle; some anticancer drugs are given by IM injection.
Intravenous (IV)	Into a vein; anticancer drugs are often given by IV injection or infusion.
Lumpectomy	Excision of a breast tumor with a limited amount of associated tissue.
Lymph Nodes	Part of the lymphatic system that removes wastes from body tissue and carries fluids that help the body fight infection. Lymph nodes in the axilla (armpit) are those most likely to be invaded by cancer cells and therefore are frequently removed during treatment for breast cancer.
Lymphedema	Swelling in the patient's arm caused by excess fluid that collects when the lymph nodes and vessels are removed during surgery or damaged by x-ray. The patient's arm and hand become more prone to infection.
Malignant Tumor	Cancerous. A growth of cancer cells. (See definition of Cancer.)
Mammography	The process of x-raying the breast to detect tumors before they can be felt.
Mastectomy	Surgical removal of the breast and some surrounding tissue for treatment of breast cancer.
Mastectomy, Modified Radical	The most common mastectomy performed today. Also called total mastectomy with axillary dissection. The breast, breast skin, nipple, areola, and underarm lymph nodes are removed, while the chest muscles are saved.
Mastectomy, Partial or Segmental	Breast surgery in which only a portion of the breast is removed, including the cancer and a surrounding margin of breast tissue.
Mastectomy Prophylactic	A procedure sometimes recommended for patients at very high risk of developing cancer in one or both breasts. One type, called a "subcutaneous" mastectomy, removes the breast tissue but leaves muscle, skin, and nipple.
Mastectomy, Radical	The surgical removal of the breast, breast skin, nipple, areola, chest muscles, and underarm lymph nodes. This operation leaves a hollow area in the chest wall under the collarbone and in front of the armpit.

Mastectomy, Simple	Breast surgery involving complete removal of the breast but not the lymph nodes or chest muscles.
Metastases	Cancer growths in one part of the body that started from cancer cells from another part.
Metastasis	Action during which cancer cells break from their original site and spread through the body.
Oncologist	A physician trained to treat patients who have cancer.
Palpation	Examining with the hand.
Pathologist	A doctor who studies cells and tissues to determine if a disease is present.
Pectoral Muscles	Muscles that overlay the chest wall and help to support the breasts.
Radiation Therapy	The use of high-energy x-rays to treat cancer.
Recurrence	Reappearance of cancer at the same site (local, near the initial site [regional], or in other areas of the body [metastatic]).
Red Blood Cells	Cells that supply oxygen to tissues throughout the body.
Remission	The disappearance of signs and symptoms of disease.
Silicone Gel	Medical grade silicone rubber gel that is similar to the fluid qualities of the normal breast.
Stomatitis	Sores on the inside lining of the mouth.
Thermography	A technique in which heat from the breast is measured and recorded. Increased temperature in one breast may indicate an abnormal condition.
Tumor	Abnormal growth of tissue.
White Blood Cells	The blood cells responsible for fighting infection.
Xeroradiography	A form of mammography that records the picture of the breast on paper, rather than on film.
X-rays	High-energy radiation used in high doses to treat cancer or in low doses to diagnose the disease.

ORGANIZATIONS AND PROGRAMS OFFERING SERVICES TO THE CANCER PATIENT AND THE FAMILY

NATIONAL ORGANIZATION
American Cancer Society Telephone: (212) 599-3600
261 Madison Avenue   Toll Free: (800) 422-6237 (days)
New York, NY 10016   Toll Free: (800) 638-6694 (eves)

General Description
Voluntary organization offering programs of cancer research, education and patient service and rehabilitation.

Psychological and Emotional Support; Education
Programs to support psychological and physical rehabilitation of patients.
Patient education and information.
Self-help and support groups in some regions.
Special programs for children and adolescents with cancer available in some regions.

Medical Physical, Logistical Support
Equipment loans for care of homebound, blood programs, surgical dressings.
Transportation to and from treatment, e.g., volunteer drivers.

Financial and Employment Assistance
Financial resource information.
Assistance with employment problems.
Temporary housing for patients near treatment centers.
Assists individuals with information on legal rights, information and education for employers, referral to vocational training.

Affiliates of The American Cancer Society, NY
*CAN SURMOUNT PROGRAM:
Composed of patient, family member, trained volunteer (also a cancer patient), health professional.
Volunteers visit hospitals and homes.
Patient and family education and information.
Personal visits.

*I CAN COPE PROGRAM:
Program that addresses the educational needs of cancer patients and their families.
Information on therapy, treatment, side effects, nutrition.
Referral to local resources.

*INTERNATIONAL ASSOCIATION OF LARYNGECTOMEES:
Voluntary umbrella organization that promotes and supports rehabilitation programs for laryngectomees.
Support and education programs for persons who have had laryngectomys.
Volunteers visit patients.
Assistance with employment adjustment on an individual basis.

*REACH TO RECOVERY PROGRAM:
Provides rehabilitation support for women who have had breast cancer.
Psychological support.
Volunteers visit hospitals.
Provide temporary prosthesis when needed.

NATIONAL ORGANIZATION
Cancer Care, Inc. Telephone: (212) 221-3300
1180 Avenue of the Americas
New York, NY 10036

General Description
The service arm of the National Cancer Foundation, a not-for-profit nonsectarian, social service agency dedicated to help patients and families cope with the emotional, psychological, and financial consequences of cancer.
Services are available at all stages of the illness.

Phychological and Emotional Support; Education
Home visits by trained volunteers.
Individual, family and group counseling to provide psychological and social support.
Literature, information and referral to local and regional resources.

Medical, Physical, Logistical Support
Develops home care plans including identifying resources

and facilitation of their implemention, e.g., health aides, housekeepers, nursing care, etc.

Financial and Employment Assistance
Work site advocacy.
Financial assistance for non-medical expenses at all stages of the disease.

NATIONAL ORGANIZATIONS
Cancer Information Service Telephone: 1-800-4-CANCER
Hawaii: Oahu (from neighbor
  islands, call collect) 524-1234
Alaska: 1-800-638-6070

General Description
A program of The National Cancer Institute consisting of a network of regional information offices that provide accurate personalized answers to cancer-related questions from patients, families, the general public, and health professionals.

Psychological and Emotional Support; Education
National Cancer Institute publications.
Trained staff and volunteers provide confidential answers to cancer-related questions.

Medical, Physical, Logistical Support
Information and referral to local and regional resources.

Financial and Employment Assistance
Information and referral to local and regional resources.

NATIONAL ORGANIZATION
Candlelighters Childhood Cancer Foundation, Inc.
2025 I Street, NW., Suite 1011
Washington, DC 20006
Telephone: (202) 659-5136

General Description
An international organization of parents whose children or adolescents have or have had cancer. Seeks to provide guidance and emotional support for families as well as

identify needs and serve as intermediary to other resources.
Patients up to age 22 are eligible for services.

Psychological and Emotional Support; Education
Self-help and support groups.
Literature, information and referral to local and regional resources.
Adolescent support groups and youth newsletter.

Medical, Physical, Logistical Support
Blood and wig banks, crisis intervention, housing near treatment centers, babysitting, transportation and other services.

Financial and Employment Assistance
Some groups provide financial assistance.

NATIONAL ORGANIZATION
CHUMS (Cancer Hopefuls United for Mutual Support)
600 West 239th Street
Riverdale, NY 10563
Telephone: (212) 796-3591

General Description
An organization of cancer survivors offering hope and emotional support to improve the quality of life for the cancer patient involving therapeutic aid through self-help, crisis intervention, information, and peer support to patients and families.

Psychological and Emotional Support; Education
Cancer survivors with similar diagnosis contact patients to provide counseling.
Support groups.
Information and referral.

Financial and Employment Assistance
Advocates of fight against employment discrimination.

NATIONAL ORGANIZATION
The Concern for Dying
250 West 57th Street, Room 831
New York, NY 10107
Telephone: (212) 246-6962

General Description
Nonprofit educational organization distributes the living will, a document that records patient wishes concerning treatment.

Psychological and Emotional Support; Education
Information regarding the living will, euthanasia, death and dying.
Psychological and legal counseling.
Referral to local organizations for other types of assistance.

NATIONAL ORGANIZATION
Corporate Angel Network
Westchester County Airport, Bldg. 1
White Plains, NY 10604
Telephone: (914) 328-1313

General Description
An organization which seeks to alleviate costs for cancer patients receiving specialized treatment in NCI-approved treatment centers by arranging transportation aboard corporate aircraft on routine flights when seats are available.

Psychological and Emotional Support; Education
Seeks to boost morale by making travel easier.

Medical, Physical, Logistical Support
Locates flights when available and arranges for ambulatory patient and one attendant or family member to fly free with U.S. corporations volunteering empty seats.

NATIONAL ORGANIZATION
Leukemia Society of America
733 Third Avenue
New York, NY 10017
Telephone: (212) 573-8484

General Description
An organization which offers financial assistance and consultation services for referrals to other means of local support to patients with leukemia and other allied disorders.

Psychological and Emotional Support; Education
Support groups for patients and families.

Financial and Employment Assistance
Financial assistance to outpatients for drugs, laboratory costs associated with transfusions, transportation, and radiation therapy.

NATIONAL ORGANIZATION
*Make-a-Wish Foundation of America
4601 North 16th Street, Suite 205
Phoenix, AZ 85016
Telephone: (602) 234-0960

General Description
A foundation which works closely with the family to grant special wishes for terminally ill children up to the age of 18.

Psychological and Emotional Support; Education
Provides special memories, encouragement, and respite from current situation by granting a special wish to a terminally ill child.

Medical, Physical, Logistical Support
Arranges for all the details involved in granting the wish. Transportation provided if it is part of a wish.

Financial and Employment Assistance
Covers all expenses incurred as a result of granting the wish.

NATIONAL ORGANIZATION
*Make Today Count
P.O. Box 222
Osage Beach, MO 65065
Telephone: (314) 348-1619

General Description
An international organization which brings together patients with cancer or other life-threatening illnesses and their families to provide a positive self-help approach to coping with a serious illness and the resulting changes in lifestyles that illness often requires.

Psychological and Emotional Support; Education
Support groups.
Education programs.

Medical, Physical, Logistical Support
Assists in communication with health professionals.

NATIONAL ORGANIZATION
National Hospice Organization
1901 North Fort Myer Drive, Suite 902
Arlington, VA 22209
Telephone: (703) 243-5900

General Description
A nonprofit membership organization consisting of groups providing hospice care; institutions concerned with care of the terminally ill and their families.

Psychological and Emotional Support; Education
Literature, information and referral to local hospice programs, and regional and national resources.

Medical, Physical, Logistical Support
Literature, information and referral to local hospice programs, and regional and national resources.

Financial and Employment Assistance
Hospice career placement listing service.

NATIONAL ORGANIZATION
United Ostomy Association
36 Executive Park, Suite 120
Irvine, CA 92714
Telephone: (714) 660-8624

General Description
Nonprofit organization with the goal to provide abdominal ostomy patients with mutual aid, moral support, and education.

Psychological and Emotional Support; Education
Members visit patients in hospitals.

Publishes quarterly magazine for members of patient education.
Provides speakers about ostomys to community groups.
Peer support groups.
Publishes patient educational booklets.

Medical, Physical, Logistical Support
Promotes better ostomy management techniques.
Encourages development of better equipment and supplies.

Financial and Employment Assistance
Insurance programs for members.
Others in progress.

REGIONAL ORGANIZATION
TOUCH
513 Tinsley Harrison Tower
University Station
Birmingham, AL 35294
Telephone: (205) 934-3814

General Description
Support groups provide assistance to cancer patients and their families in forming realistic, positive attitudes toward cancer and its treatment.

Psychological and Emotional Support; Education
Counselors provide peer emotional support for in- and out-patients.
Continuing education on treatment methods.

REGIONAL ORGANIZATION
We Can Do!
P.O. Box 723
Arcadia, CA 91006
Telephone: (818) 357-7517

General Description
A support program that addresses the long-term psychological and educational needs of cancer patients, cancer survivors, and family members.

Psychological and Emotional Support; Education
Support groups meet weekly on a continuing basis (California and Washington, D.C. only)
Educational programs.
Referral to local resources.
Classes for spouses of cancer patients.

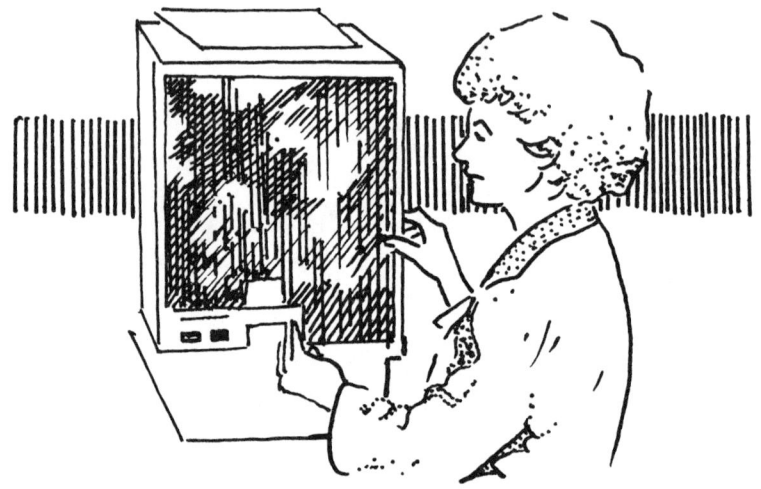

If you care to comment or make any suggestions on this writing, please feel free to do so. Send all correspondence to Aurora Publishing Co., P.O. Box 2537, Garden City, Kansas 67846. If you wish additional copies you may call our toll free number 1-800-535-5111.

Thank you very much and

                                          Good Health!

                                    Dr. Paul Rodriguez

NOTES

NOTES

NOTES

NOTES

NOTES

NOTES